a call
to
nursing

a call
to
nursing

Stories about
Challenge and
Commitment

Paula Sergi, BSN, MFA
Geraldine Gorman, RN, PhD
Editors

KAPLAN PUBLISHING

New York

This publication is designed to provide accurate and authoritative information in regard to the subject matter covered. It is sold with the understanding that the publisher is not engaged in rendering medical or other professional service. If medical advice or other expert assistance is required, the services of a competent professional should be sought.

While the stories in *A Call to Nursing* are based on real events, names, places, and other details have been changed for the sake of privacy.

Published by Kaplan Publishing, a division of Kaplan, Inc.
1 Liberty Plaza, 24th Floor
New York, NY 10006

Printed in the United States of America

10 9 8 7 6 5 4 3

Library of Congress Cataloging-in-Publication Data

A call to nursing : nurses' stories about challenge and commitment / Paula M. Sergi, Geraldine Gorman, editors.
    p. ; cm.
    Includes bibliographical references and index.
    ISBN 978-1-4277-9863-3 (alk. paper)
    1. Nursing—Anecdotes. 2. Nurses' writings, American. 3. Vocation. 4. Commitment (Psychology) I. Sergi, Paula, 1952- II. Gorman, Geraldine.
    [DNLM: 1. Nurses—psychology—Personal Narratives. 2. Nurse-Patient Relations—Personal Narratives. 3. Nursing—Personal Narratives. WY 87 C156 2009]
    RT34.C35 2009
    610.73—dc22

                                 2008053899

Kaplan Publishing books are available at special quantity discounts to use for sales promotions, employee premiums, or educational purposes. Please email our Special Sales Department to order or for more information at *kaplanpublishing@kaplan.com*, or write to Kaplan Publishing, 1 Liberty Plaza, 24th Floor, New York, NY 10006.

Contents

Introduction

TIME'S PASSAGE "FROM one summer to the next [is] marked by noting a single memorable event." So nurse-poet Veneta Masson reminds us in her evocative litany, "Winter Count." A brief encounter with a patient, a conversation with a friend, or another seemingly chance encounter can change the course of our lives — or our careers. Occasionally, these experiences serve as epiphanies, flashes of knowledge, that guide as we move forward.

As a practice profession, nursing abounds with experiences that can either reinforce our vocational commitment or cause us to reconsider it. It is not uncommon to encounter both such mindsets, sometimes in the course of a single day. For many of us, the demands of the profession and the deeply personal and intimate nature of our relationships with people cause us to question whether we are in the right place. How we face such moments, whether we recommit ourselves or decide to leave, determines not only the trajectory of our lives but the tapestry of the profession.

This collection gathers stories from nurses in all phases of their careers — past and present — who stood within such life-changing moments and emerged from them with new understanding about themselves and their professions.

The book is divided into three parts. The first section, *The Calling*, offers the idealistic reflections of those aglow with nursing's promise of intimacy and connection. In *Bus Ride, Away Game*, writer, poet and practicing ER nurse Jeanne Bryner describes how the work of her hands shaped her narrative:

> I went home tired, my heart's pockets full, bulging with stories of hope, grief and giving. Here were the hallways of sleepy or cranky voices. The hands and calloused feet fit for poetry stanzas. Here was the embryonic room of my inner library, a place to catalog hard telling moments which make us rich.

In the second part, *The Reckoning*, writers share the deep reservations endemic to the clash of idealism and reality. Nursing is often not what we expected. We are then forced to learn to cope or to leave the profession. In *Supreme Love and Caring*, nurse and musician Colleen O'Brien tells how music "has become a life source, a treasure, a sublime sanity in this world that lately has seemed so insane. It is a place (of supreme love and caring) for connection of heart, mind and soul and for connection with others." It saved her from the burnout of years in nursing.

Try as she might, Jenna Rindo never felt comfortable with making that kind of connection in clinical settings. Instead, she always felt the outsider, watching those native to the terrain: "I would listen to lung sounds again and again. Did I hear subtle crackles in the lower left lung lobe? How could those lips look slightly cyanotic when the Pulse Ox clearly read 97%? Seasoned nurses develop a sixth sense when something doesn't look or feel right about a patient. I perceived them as having some sort of special power to foresee and then ward off a patient crash or crisis that I felt I clearly lacked." Clearly, the time had come to move on.

The final section, *The Promise,* expresses the commitment that arises only after sustained trial. As with any valued relationship, such renewal of vows can occur after 40 years of practice or after 3 months of apprenticeship. Intimate knowledge can breed contempt or deepen wonder. Poet-turned-nursing student Shirley Stephenson considers the memorable events she has encountered thus far. Her affirmative response: "I'm Staying" forms a celebratory litany of ambiguity:

> Because there is no map and way to pack for certain journeys . . . . Because the bedside tray and the call button become the whole world. Because wisdom, grace and ferocity hibernate in each tired body. Because even when thumping, the heart is fragile.

Whether you are a nurse reflecting on the moments that marked seasonal passage through your career or you are a fellow traveler who faced the reckoning of intimate encounter and took a stand, we believe the voices gathered here will speak to you, as they continue to resonate for us.

Paula Sergi
Geraldine Gorman

a call to nursing

PART ONE

The Calling

*Reflections of nurses aglow with
nursing's promise of intimacy*

Grounding

~

Anita Chupp, RN

I HAVEN'T TOLD MANY people this—in fact, I think I have only told one—but nursing is my calling. I embrace this feeling even if I am embarrassed by it. It is not logical or scientific. It is a sentiment related to spirituality, and even the word *spirituality* seems to make people uneasy. I certainly could not have written in my application essay for the University of Illinois College of Nursing that one of the qualities I would bring to the nursing profession is a profound sense of calling. Truth be told, I do not even know who or what is calling me—an ethereal being floating above me in fluffy white clouds; Mother Nature, whose cold breath chills me on morning walks with the dog; or some other source, like powered magnets? It seems silly that anyone or anything would make the effort to tell one person what her professional endeavor should be. All I am banking on at the moment is that there is something sitting inside me that allows me to question people, places, and policies, but never my desire to be a nurse.

I am grounded in this feeling that I say is my calling. It is a secret I cannot adequately convey to the people I love most, because I do not have words to describe the surge of electricity that shoots up my spine when I, as a student nurse, take part in the process of healing. I cannot explain the sheer sense of panic I feel when I read about all the different shades and colors of health disparities in our world; I get overwhelmed and feel like there are too many causes to choose from. I do not yet have enough knowledge, but something in my gut rumbles when I see the need people have for advocates in our healthcare system. It is this feeling of being called to serve, care, and advocate that pulls my eyelids open at the crack of dawn to put on my ciel blue polyester-blend scrubs with the UIC College of Nursing emblem that tells the world, or at the very least the oncology floor of the medical center, that I am a student nurse.

Of course, being a neophyte nursing student is not all idealistic whimsy. My skin crawls when I am told that I am, in the hierarchy that is healthcare, the low man on the totem pole—that is a terrible phrase, and I am a woman! My cheeks blaze when a staff nurse tells me to give a bed bath to a 73-year-old female patient while two hulking young male physical therapists are working with her weak and wasting limbs. I hate the residents for not looking me in the eye when they pass me in the hall or stand next to me over a patient's bed. I loathe the system that pushes barely recovered people out the door, and pushes especially hard if they don't have insurance.

And those reactions and feelings don't even take into account the nursing-school part. I spend most of my waking hours either trying to cram as much information as I can into my brain or feeling guilty that I am doing something other than cramming as much information as possible into my brain.

I am living, breathing, and sleeping nursing; I can barely think of anything else. The patients I had for two days occupy my mind for the rest of the week. I wonder about ways to incorporate other modalities of healing into the field of nursing. I wonder if there is a way that everyone can benefit from preventive healthcare for the poor. And I am still working on convincing the man that I love that giving injections is really cool.

Danger: Student Nurse

~

Kelly Fitzgerald

I'M GOING TO murder someone. Someone's grandmother. Someone's mother. Someone's husband. Someone's
sister. When I get to the clinical setting next month, I am
going to fuck up royally and someone is going to die. You
should watch for me on the evening news. I'll be wearing big
white clogs. My proud parents have TiVo, so if you miss the
story at ten o'clock, give them a call; my stepfather can fill
you in on my criminal activity. Growing up, I listened to my
parents' horror stories about staffers accidentally murdering
patients at the teaching hospital they both worked in. My
favorite (the one I found to be most terrifying) was the one
about the resident who diagnosed pulmonary edema with
the patient's X-ray turned around. He inserted the needle
to drain the wrong lung; it collapsed, and the patient died.
When I was 14 years old, the internist treating my grandfather failed to order intake and output monitoring when his

kidney function was compromised. Cause of death: complications from acute renal failure. In our house, it is common knowledge that Andy Warhol died because his private-duty nurse failed to empty his catheter bag.

Now I am the professional who might one day mess up somebody's care. According to the college of nursing I attend and Mount Sinai Hospital, I am ready for contact with human patients with genuine ailments. This conclusion is based on the fact that I've kept up with the reading and passed my skills evaluations each week. That qualifies me to care for patients? I can't even care for myself: I go weeks at a time without shaving my legs, I have enormous credit card debt, and I frequently skip breakfast.

I know that there will be a clinical supervisor on-site and that each patient already has an assigned RN. I am merely an accessory. I will be watched like a hawk, they assure me. What if they don't watch me closely enough? After all, there is a nursing shortage in this country! What if my clinical supervisor goes to the bathroom and a lazy RN delegates her work to me—and I give Mr. Smith's intravenous dose of Versed to Mrs. Jones orally? What mechanism is in place to keep me from losing a Q-tip deep into the sinus tract of Mr. Johnson's pressure ulcer? Who will make sure I don't trip on a dangling tube and rip out Ms. Williams's central line? I cannot be trusted!

All I know is that I must make a conscious effort to reduce Kelly Fitzgerald–related patient mortality. I will stay close to my clinical instructor. I will not leave her side. If she does try to escape to the bathroom, I will hold her lab coat for her outside the stall. I will not be made to do the lazy

RN's work. I will read the medication order at least three times while preparing the medication. I will write the name of the medication on a sheet of scrap paper. I will read it aloud to the rest of my clinical group, at least two RNs, and someone from risk management. I will make up an easy-to-remember song about it. I will regularly review my textbooks, familiarizing myself with my patients' diseases. I will get eight hours of sleep each night. I will eat a well-balanced breakfast each morning. I will not murder a patient. I will not murder a patient. I will not murder a patient . . . .

Bus Ride,
Away Game, 1968

~

Jeanne Bryner, RN, BA, CEN

In BLISSFUL IGNORANCE children believe, however briefly, that all avenues are open to them and that education may be possible with enormous effort. We all aspire to "be somebody"—Diana Ross, Ginger Rogers, Katharine Hepburn—and self-actualization becomes a ladder that keeps unfolding on our journey. At 16, I was no different. Raised in a family with six children (my youngest brother had cerebral palsy) and ailing parents (Mother suffered from manic depression, Father was an alcoholic), I learned early on to survive: we had to circle the wagons of our bodies around the campfires of our minds.

Taking care of others is as natural as breathing to me, and whether my vocation would come under the label of nurse's aide, physical therapist, or nurse was a mystery to be figured out in the fog's distance. The winds of time carry family seeds. For me, my mother and granny mentioned on several occasions that I had "good hands" and would make "a pretty nurse like Aunt Thelma's girl." Of course, as a kid, I enjoyed hearing these comments while I rubbed cold cream on Granny's tired face. Suffering from mental illness, Mother spent more time in the hospital getting electroshock therapy than at home. I would have gladly cut off my fingers, one at a time with a dull knife, to bring her even a moment of happiness.

Before I was nine years old, Father divorced his sick wife, my mother. Her illness blew her ragged, and like a kite she was accepted in the branches of family homes. My grandparents' West Virginia farm seemed her favorite branch. Some summers we visited her there; but the time we shared was strained, for our visits usually triggered a manic phase. As a child, you believe it's all your fault. Maybe you needed to be quieter, more polite, and then she'd be like the other mothers who moved through their head-scarf-over-pin-curls days cooking meatloaf, cleaning bathtubs, and speaking monotone sentences. All my life, I saw my friends with their mothers who were well and, I believed, happy. So, to me, sadness and sickness were two sides to the same pillow, and that pillow smothered my mother's face.

Then one spring day she had a seizure and went into a coma; she died within a week. At her funeral, my sister leaned close to ask me, "Doesn't it make you want to be a nurse more than ever?" I was so overcome with Mother's passing that I could barely nod. It was five days after my high school graduation and five days before my 18th birthday.

After the funeral, my uncle, her brother, was suffering so greatly that I had to drive his entire family back to Ohio. Nobody seemed to know why Mother had died. She had no history of seizures. What had happened? Reluctantly, my grandparents agreed to an autopsy. They were going to "cut her open;" somehow they were trying to pry secrets from the tomb of her body. The report was inconclusive for the cause of death.

All of this happened a year and a half after a bus ride I took to an away football game. The cheerleaders sat together as the bus made its way to the game. I was the school mascot, the tiger. Who knows how one teenage girl talks to another about life goals? Are the words a form of divine providence or just small talk to fill the darkness? It was the autumn of my junior year, and Margo Macauley and I were chatting about Cher Bono's blue eye shadow, hot-pink rib ticklers, and Margo's plan to become a registered nurse. Margo was a bubbly sandy-haired girl with freckle dust sprinkled across her nose and a warm, easy smile. As I recall the conversation through the lens of memory, it went something like this:

I'm going to live at the dorm in nurse's training, but it's just in Warren.
What do you have to take to get into nursing?
One unit each of chemistry, biology, and algebra.
Huh. No Latin?
No Latin.
But I thought you had to take Latin.
Nope.

Well, I only have one year left, and I haven't had any of those sciences.

There's summer school.

But I waitress.

It's only half a day.

All summer?

Nope.

What about the new chemistry teacher? He's so fat and sweaty.

They say he's nice, you know, not as cranky as old Mr. Bauer.

Oh yeah?

Yeah.

I'm not very good at math.

Algebra's not hard.

Really?

Really.

Say I take chemistry next summer. Then what?

You sign up for algebra and biology for your senior year.

I guess I could try. What else do you have to do?

A physical, some tests—you know—the ACT, SAT, and NLN.

(I did not know.) Well, I've been taking business classes. I don't like them, but it's what Kathy (my best friend) takes. I can't even read my own shorthand back in class. (We both laughed.)

Go to the guidance office. There are forms, dates, locations for testing. Talk to Mr. Hudsin.

He seems so goofy.

You have to.

That NLN thing—what's that?

It's a National League for Nursing test. You have to do it.

Have you?

Yep.

And how was it?

Study up on your vocabulary.

Vocab? Really?

Yep. Reading is important. Any field you choose, you gotta be able to read and understand.

Want some gum?

Yep.

For nursing school, how much?

Cheaper than four years of college.

Really?

Yep. My folks are paying for my sister Lynn, so you know.

Yeah, where are you going?

Right here in Warren, Trumbull Memorial Hospital School of Nursing. It's close.

Really?

Yep. I already visited the school, dorms, and hospital with my folks.

And?

The rooms are small, but it's close to home and affordable. The school's good. I just remembered—you have to see a dentist.

Why?

I don't know. It's part of it. Just take the papers
with you when you go.

I'D NEVER SEEN a dentist in my life. Never had a tooth-
ache. I thought that's the only reason a person went to the
dentist. In our family, only my sister went. She had "soft
teeth," and, that being her curse, she got cavities. Two years
older than me, she came home with horror stories about our
town dentist and the blood smeared across his white smock.
Everything attached to healing and wellness seemed frightening; still, I wanted my ticket for that smoky train.

And summer-school chemistry turned out not to be a
torment. Robbie Campbell caught her sink on fire during
the first experiment, and that let us know this was serious business. The Vietnam War raged across the oceans,
the Kennedy brothers lay dead, and Robbie Campbell sat
right behind me. How foolish to think there's any safe
place. After the fire I made sure to wear my long hair in
a ponytail. Meanwhile, the fat, sweaty chemistry teacher
turned out to be a human being who saw how I struggled
to balance equations without any algebraic knowledge; with
the powers of the gods, he gave me a blessed C– for the
course. What he didn't know was how I struggled on the
tightrope that stretched between school and home. Father
was between wives, my sisters were off to California, and so
I was in charge of my brothers and the house. The hallowed
halls of Domestica held me close.

In biology that fall, my partner was a bright 15-year-old
Catholic boy named Jack. He'd go on to pitch his heart out at

Miami University, winning our state's college baseball title. The first day of class, I remember the teacher, Mr. Russell, saying how it showed maturity for a senior (me) to partner with a freshman. I can still smell the formaldehyde on our fumbling hands and hear the birdsong playing on the black records for us to identify.

Algebra was not the boulder I had imagined, and I found out that how the subject is explained makes all the difference. My teacher was a woman, an angel truly. She took me by the hand and demystified the negative space of those equations.

I passed all the tests I needed to get into nurses' training, but my piggybank held no money when it was time for tuition. The local factory was hiring lots of high school graduates to build wiring harnesses for automobiles. It was there I landed a job that had insurance, retirement, and vacation. Six months after graduating from high school, I had left home, secured an apartment, been laid off, and married a man with a five-year-old son. Over the next two and a half years I would be called back and forth to work at the factory. Finally, I "retired early" and enrolled in a cake-decorating class with my still best friend, Kathy. We made exceptionally beautiful roses, and for a while those birthday/first-holy-communion/wedding cakes helped fill my hungry days.

Still longing to be a nurse, I made saving for my education a priority. The autumn I was to start at Youngstown State University, our furnace blew up. We went to plan B, and our savings provided a dandy new furnace. Without knowing Maslow's hierarchy of needs, we lived it, placing our most basic needs first.

By the time the moon and stars and planets lined up correctly for nursing education, I was 25 years old. Almost the old lady of the 1976 class, I plunged headfirst into a world of 22 hours of course work the first quarter, 21 hours the second quarter, and so on. The reading pressed me to a secluded room upstairs, and my husband (bless him) took over nearly all of Domestica.

Though I had never been a candy striper or any other type of hospital volunteer, from the first day of clinicals I knew I was born for nursing. As I bathed an elderly patient or held an emesis basin for a surgical patient or figured doses for a child's pain shot, I thought, *This is what I've been doing all of my life; now I'm going to get a paycheck for it.* I went home tired, my heart's pockets full, bulging with stories of hope, grief, and giving. Here were the hallways of sleepy or cranky voices, the bandaged hands and callused feet fit for poetry stanzas. Here was the embryonic room of my inner library, a place to catalog the hard, telling moments that make us rich.

My school nurse, Lois Laidig, was and is a special person. Always I admired her quiet confidence and sought her counsel when I was considering nursing, but it's Margo Macauley I must thank for the trinity of chemistry, biology, and algebra. It's her voice I hear again, above the Juicy Fruit and the hum of those big bus tires, as I sift and decipher this road's graveled back. Without our little chat on the yellow bus, I might still be moving on the factory line.

If you look at the documentation, you'll see that for more than a quarter of a century I've been a practicing nurse. If you study my life, the time can be doubled. I have never dreaded going to work, and that is a blessing. People are amazing and genuine in all their complexities. When people are part of the problem, there is no equation, no predictability. I like that most of all. No formula works. A quilt of faces appears: who we are, what we can do, all sorts of patterns and colors. Sometimes a gentle thread slips between women in pivotal moments, and that thread may be connected to monastic bells. I grow quiet remembering, listening, giving thanks.

From Things Unspecific

~

Lise Kunkel, RN

Split wide open, midline peeled back,
Tissue yellow-gray,
Fluids pool in the distal portion.
She lies flat,
A series of tubes to gravity,
Hairless from chemo.

I irrigate, flushing sanguineous ponds
From the belly of her wound.
She is sleeping.
Lashless, thin like phyllo dough,
Her eyelids make sleeping movements,
Her wide Dutch features still.

She is very young.
It is spring.
They are standing on a hill overlooking the lake.
He tells her she is lovely.
She smiles full-toothed—
Cheeks flushed, eyes effulgent, she breaks into a run.

I collect her fluids in a graduated cylinder,
Adjust the dressings, check the tubes.
Reaching for the bed light, I touch
Her smooth skull, trace the bone
Down her cheekline.
Sixty years of expression accepts
My brief passage.

"Katherine, you are beautiful," I tell her.
"Yes," she replies—
in the language of silence.

Bodyguard

~

William Dineen

Sometimes when i am in the hospital as a student nurse, I feel that I actually have a career as a personal assistant/bodyguard to a famous recluse. Student nurses have a luxury that regular floor nurses don't: we take care of no more than one or two patients at a time. I have the opportunity to leisurely provide morning care, change the bed linens, and then give each patient a soothing, moisturizing massage. Due to staffing shortages nationwide, most nurses are pulled in many different directions at any one time, with five or more patients clamoring for their attention. One nurse even cautioned me to warn my patients not to get used to the royal treatment because when the students went back to class, spa time was over!

If there is one thing I have never been able to tolerate, it's too many cooks in the kitchen. In my previous career as a law enforcement officer, I could never understand why every cop on duty had to run over to the scene of an incident when just one or two officers could easily handle the situation. Even the individuals involved in whatever it was, be it a domestic incident or an auto accident, deserved a bit of privacy at a time that clearly wasn't optimal. I still operate that way as a student nurse. I tend to keep the door closed and, like a loyal bulldog, viciously protect my patients' privacy and dignity. While it's great that floor staff check in with the "new kid," how much assistance do I really need to change linens or do morning care on a fairly independent patient? Worse is how many times, while trying to bathe my patient, I have had to shut the door behind the doctor or nurse who left it wide open! Does this sick person really need to hear every page in the hallway or every clang of gurneys and hum of floor polishers? Sometimes I just want to scream in my best New York cabbie voice, "Hey! We're healing over here!! Can ya hold it down?"

Yes, it's true. I feel very protective of my patients. I spoil them a bit, and justifiably so. Patients never have to take on a student nurse; they have the right to demand a fully licensed nurse should they so desire. I am grateful for the opportunity to work my craft, practice my nursing skills, and develop the fine art of establishing a therapeutic relationship. Each female patient is like a mother or sister to me; each male, my compatriot brother. Of course I am going to protect them, but I also protect myself in the process. I am protecting myself from the inevitable development of faster, better skills; from having been licensed; from caring for too many patients at a time, being pulled in all directions, needing to just go to the washroom and not being able to find time!

I relish this time with my patients. I treasure the legacy of my foremothers who lovingly cared for soldiers with no supplies, few comforts, and even less knowledge about disease. It wasn't about how many or how much or who was going to pay for it all. It was about that magical time when a nurse touches the heart of a patient and an authentic connection, a healing moment, is made.

My Many Mentors

~

Joan Stack Kovach, RN, MS, PC

W HEN I WAS three years old, I swallowed a nickel—
not just any nickel, but one from my oldest brother's miniature jukebox bank. The story that remains, and that may
have some resemblance to some truth, is that one day I was
sent up to take my nap in Billy's room. There, instead of falling asleep, I explored the contents of his shelves. Intrigued
by his beautiful red marbled-plastic jukebox bank, I shook
it up and down until a nickel fell out. At this point I heard
my mother approaching and quickly hid the nickel in my
mouth. I don't recall anything else until a lunchtime scene
later that day, or maybe a few days after. I was giving the dog
my leftover chicken noodle soup, because I couldn't swallow
it. I was the fourth in a family of ten children, so it took
something special for my mother to decide there needed to
be a visit to the doctor. This—a three-year-old not swallow-
ing, giving her favorite soup to the dog—qualified.

The next memory I have is of being on a rolling bed, entering an elevator with an accordion folding door. There, a nurse with white shoes and stockings told me to look at the monkey perched up in the far corner of the elevator. Then I fell asleep. When I awoke, my throat was sore and my mother (or was it the nurse?) was tying up my high shoes so that I could go home. After that, my mother kept an ugly greenish nickel in a tiny cardboard earring box in her top dresser drawer. It was said to be "the nickel Joanie swallowed." My sister Jeania did not believe the part about the monkey, and she teased me about it.

Another scene from my memory took place 14 years later. Jeania had come home from college for Thanksgiving. Glad for a chance to escape the noise and hubbub of our home, she and I eagerly agreed to go out to pick up some more milk. We drove the mile to an outdoor vending machine, where in those days a quarter bought a quart of milk.

Now that I had her alone, I asked about college. She was a freshman at Niagara University School of Nursing. She told me about the girls in her dorm, the new shampoos she had tried, the prolific use of sunlamps, and the Indian chemistry professor who wailed "Oh no, not the lamp!" when girls showed up for class beet red from the artificial sunburn. These are the specifics I remember, but somewhere in there probably was woven the inspiration to follow in her footsteps and become a nurse. At any rate there was the evidence that leaving home and studying something was a great liberating adventure. All my life I had used the same shampoo (Lustre Crème, a pearly pink substance in professional-size jars big enough for a goldfish), and that was long enough. Now I was hearing that life holds excitement, freedom, and choices—and that I too could be a nurse.

In 1965, I was thinking about college, thinking about liking biology and maybe trying to be a doctor. But I was also thinking that I wanted to be a mother, and I knew no doctors who were mothers, only ones like our family doctor, who sent me to Nyack Hospital to have the nickel removed, and then his son, a second-generation family doctor who did my sports physical each year so I could be a cheerleader. They both had dedicated wives taking care of everything else in their lives so that they could be there for my four brothers and five sisters and me, their patients. So I began to think again about nursing.

In 1966, I entered nursing school at Georgetown University. I finished in 1970, began a master's program in psychiatric nursing in 1972, and received my master's degree in 1974, all the while not knowing who or what was guiding me, helping me make those most excellent choices, ones I have never regretted.

Amid that time, in 1971, my mother—57 years young, ripe enough to be thinking about collecting some Social Security soon, all ten kids nearly raised and gone and a half dozen foster kids in and out of her home as well—signed up for an associate's degree program in nursing at the community college. With sheer persistence and determination, she got the school to accept her credits from her short stint at a New York City college 40-plus years earlier. With this head start, she struggled through the courses and clinicals, biting her tongue as the instructor for the obstetrical nursing rotation "taught" her how to diaper a baby "the right way." At the end of the two years, she received a failing grade for her medical-surgical clinical rotation. "Someone your age will be looked upon as having a great deal of experience, as knowing more than you know right now. Perhaps you will repeat the clinical rotation and be successful in passing it the second time," her instructor told her.

We, her ten children, were appalled, especially her two nurse daughters. We rallied to her defense, suggesting an age discrimination suit. She decided instead to take advantage of the opportunity to take the LPN boards; she passed them and postponed for a while her dream of becoming an RN so she could start work as an LPN.

At first she was content with home care. On her days off, as they sat and shared lunch, she entertained my father, a retired insurance agent and school bus driver, with stories about the people she cared for and the characters she encountered in her work.

After about a year, she left home care to work at a local residential treatment center, which back then we called the orphanage. I'm not sure why she changed jobs. Perhaps she missed taking care of children. She worked in the infirmary of the orphanage, dispensing medicine to the troubled girls and boys in her care. Behind her in the nurses' station, facing her charges as they appeared at the med room door for their antiseizure, antidepressant, antibiotic, and other medications, a full-sized poster of Uncle Sam stared down. His pants had bold blue stripes, his jacket had spangled red stars, and his top hat sported both. With his right arm outstretched and his right hand pointing at whoever glanced up at him, with his severe and challenging gaze, he asked, "Have you had your pill today?" My mother—Mrs. Jean Stack the infirmary nurse, the mother of ten children and a growing brood of grandchildren—was uncomfortable under his gaze. She was uncomfortable with his message, and equally uncomfortable with the psychotropic and birth control pills she was dispensing to children so much less innocent, so much less cared about than her own were at their age. But she was not too uncomfortable to carry out her job, and carry home more stories of the children in her care, some of them twice her size, with more previous addresses than she had ever known and more foster parents than she had children.

Mom died in September 2000. I wish I could ask her now why and when she left that job. I have no doubt that those at the orphanage were sorry to lose her, even if she could not approve of so much that composed the healthcare of those kids, her second big batch of kids. She worked until the needs of her family—of grandchildren in many states wanting her company and children seeking her helpful visits—took her off the nursing schedule. And when peripheral vascular dementia arrived, and meant that she needed care, my nurse sisters took her in. We all helped, providing her with the care that she taught us about.

In 1996, three children and many jobs later, I agreed to bring a flyer to a local psychiatric nurse meeting I was attending in order to stay connected to my profession while I was mostly at home with kids. The flyer was seeking nurses to work on an evaluation team in the emergency room. This was work I had never done, only wondered at, feared actually. Counterphobically, I applied, mostly to learn more about it. I was hired, and when I asked why, my new boss, Gail, told me, "I knew I could take on one person to teach this to, and you bring other skills, so I wanted you on the team."

Teach me she did. I learned to master that which scared me most. I learned that while many devastating symptoms and debilitating disease processes cannot be fixed, they can be managed. And for five years I learned and practiced how to manage psychiatric emergencies. Another mentor had been presented to me.

Most recently, I have found myself leading an inpatient team, a team that works daily at many tasks I have not yet mastered myself. When they have questions, they ask me. And when I have no answers, I turn to my colleagues, doing the same job on other hospital units, for advice. More mentors. Just in time too.

One day as I drove to work last month, my mind only on how heavy the commute might be, traffic slowed on a stretch of road where the pace usually quickens. There was some confusion ahead: cars were pulled to the side, men in suits and ties were running across the street to the woods, and one man held a cell phone to his ear while he directed traffic. Soft gray steam or smoke was wafting up from a ditch in the woods, just off the shoulder of the road. Another car in the oncoming traffic pulled over and stopped, and then I saw her, white T-shirt, blue scrub pants, bandage scissors bouncing on her hip as she ran toward the smoke. It was another nurse in the sisterhood of nurses, driving home, I imagined, tired from her 12-hour night shift, but doing what she must: bringing her energy and her skill to the aid of a stranger. The victim by the side of the road was conscious and alert, if bloody, and had people at her side. I am not practiced in acute or emergency care. The only skills I could offer, those of a psychiatric nurse, were already being provided by others. So I moved on, knowing this auto accident victim was in good hands until the EMTs arrived.

So who can I call my mentor? Who inspired me to be a nurse? Who continues to inspire me? Those are complicated questions that demand a textured, multilayered answer.

Was it the nurse of my childhood, the one with the white shoes and stockings? My heroic and energetic sister? My legendary mother, the one who taught me first about providing care? Gail, who took such a risk to bring me into the emergency room? The other ER nurses? The nurse running on the side of the road? The psych nurse peer group I've met with monthly for 25 years? My colleagues at the hospital? The staff nurses on my unit? The nurse writers I've met and write with? Yes, I think so. They all inspire me, and we all inspire each other.

Even though I am a clinical specialist and my mother was an LPN, and even though I had my license to practice before she started back to school, she is my inspiration, mine and my sister's. I never lived in the same town with my sister after she received her nursing degree, and she practiced community health whereas I focused on mental health, but of course she inspired me. She taught me how to make my nursing practice my own, to put my personality in it, to take something from it, some joy and satisfaction each day too.

The nurses I worked side by side with in the ER scared me to death at first. They were brisk, frank, fast, sometimes sharp. Remember, I'm a psychiatric nurse. Over time I learned not only that they were bright, accurate, kind, and caring but also that they saved lives, and loved the lives they saved. They were my mentors.

The woman I saw run past me that recent morning might be 20 years younger than me, may not even have been born when I began nursing school. But she too is my mentor and inspiration, a reason to keep being a nurse, to remain in this marvelous sisterhood.

What I love about nursing is the way it legitimizes caring. In fact, I am paid to care. You can't really tell that as much now as when I started, back when risk management, malpractice insurance, cost-cutting, and managed care and its accompanying paperwork were negligible influences. Things have changed a great deal. One day in the midst of the most drastic of these changes, at a time when nurses were being abruptly fired to save money, a nurse friend said sadly, "We are the last generation of nurses paid to care." Happily, I now believe she was wrong.

I manage an acute psychiatric unit staffed by professional nurses who love their work and commit themselves wholeheartedly to it, and they too inspire me. They are not paid much, but they deliver compassionate care, safely, to the mentally ill, and they do it every day. What a privilege to work with them.

Maybe I went into nursing to find out the truth about the monkey in the elevator. I still don't know if there really was a monkey there, as my groggy preoperative preschool self firmly believed. But I know other things, and that is enough. My mentors have transcended time and place. I am grateful for all the inspirations and for all those who contributed to helping me find my place as a nurse.

Nursing Arts Manual

~

Nancy Seale Osborne, BS, MS, MLS

M_Y MOTHER WOULD have been proud of me. It took great patience for her to teach me to tie my shoes. But by the time I went to an early kindergarten at the age of four, tying my shoes had become second nature to me each morning before I reached for my lunch pail, gave Blackie a last head pat, and eagerly headed for Mrs. Fitzgerald's classroom.

Now I was learning about infection control, and the tying and untying of hospital gowns.

What should you do first when putting on a gown?

a. Tie the waist strings.
b. Tie the strings at the neck.
c. Overlap the back of the gown.
d. Make sure it completely covers all of your uniform.

The answer, it turns out, is *d,* because the sink you will be leaning against after you put on your gown is considered dirty. But to be completely covered, wouldn't you also have to overlap the back of the gown, and tie it at the waist and neck?

Mrs. Maggie McGowan was one of my third-floor postsurgical patients. She got a great kick out of the story about my being tested and retested about the donning and discarding of my hospital gown. I told her she liked the story because of her last name, and asked if she would mind if I named my hospital gown "Maggie" after her. She roared with laughter at the prospect.

My instructor in nursing arts later offered her approval of my hospital gown procedures, but she asked me to tone down my storytelling a little bit, reminding me that Mrs. McGowan's stitches hadn't yet been removed.

Why was everything so complicated? I felt a forehead. It was hot. Must be a fever. My patient told me she couldn't stop shaking. I got a blanket, stat. I wanted to record something simple on the chart, like "fever and chills," but having just completed my skills competency review, I knew that there were 15 procedures to taking a patient's temperature and that an accurate thermometer reading was paramount. I ran water in the sink and scrubbed my hands as I smiled at the patient sympathetically. Her covers to her chin, her eyes wide, she looked afraid—not of me, but of just being there in the tall hospital bed. I checked her ID bracelet and called her by name.

"Helen," I began, and she acknowledged me with an imperceptible nod. "I'm about to take your temperature and record it on your chart." She nodded again. I knew the answer to the next question, but I asked it because it was step 4 of of the section called "Measuring the Oral Temperature" in my nursing arts manual: "Have you had anything to drink or eat, or have you smoked or chewed gum, in the past 15 minutes?" If she replied in the affirmative, I would have to return later. But Helen shook her head no.

I winked and let her know that was hunky-dory, even though winking was not in the procedures, and I put my rubber gloves on, snapping them smartly. Helen jumped at the noise, and I felt chagrined that my authority, even as a nursing student, frightened a patient.

I rinsed the disinfectant solution off the thermometer and shook its mercury down below 96 degrees Fahrenheit, gently placing it under Helen's tongue. "Keep your lips around the thermometer," I suggested with a smile, gazing at my watch's minute hands for three long minutes.

After the requisite time, I read the thermometer, trying not to look alarmed at the fact that it registered very high for an adult temperature. As I recorded the temperature, I saw a small terrarium and bent over to see the tiny mosses and plants.

Helen whispered, "It's from my little boy. He's only three."

"It's magnificent, like a tiny forest," I told her, smiling. I would have loved to read her entire chart, to curl up in the chair by her and let her tell me about her son. Instead, I returned the thermometer to its container, removed my gloves, washed my hands, and told her, "Helen, I promise to you that all day long I will think about walking in a forest!" Her wan smile followed me out the door.

"MAKE SURE THAT a woman's breasts are not caught under the belt." I surmise that there are parts of a man that also would not be appropriate to confine with a transfer or gait belt. But only the woman's breasts were mentioned in our nursing arts materials. There were so many things to learn about transferring a person from bed to chair: checking ahead of time to see which is the weaker side of a person's body, watching for paleness (pallor) or blueness (cyanosis), listening for signs of dizziness or lightheadedness, watching for difficult breathing (or dyspnea). And all of this was just about the person being transferred.

"Make sure you've eaten a good breakfast. Make sure you've worked out so that your legs and back are strong. You will need to learn how to transfer from bed to wheelchair, from bed to stretcher. You will need to learn about the various positions of a person in bed, the implementation of small pillows at critical body places, the uses of small, rolled towels."

I practiced these movements and uses ad infinitum with my classmates, over popcorn and Dr Pepper, with pizza ordered late at night. I learned about repositioning limbs, transferring bodies, applying belts, and installing and removing pillows. I learned that I needed strength and stamina and gumption.

We had the notion of patients' rights drilled into us, young as we were, and I can't help but think a lot of it stuck. We never mentioned patients' names, even when we were being exceptionally goofy after a long day of classroom and on-floor duty.

At night in our dormitory rooms, we mimicked our nursing instructors, whose primary concern, beyond not getting their students killed in their daily rounds of duty, was good patient care. Our humorous escapades relieved our tension, but that behavior wasn't very nice of us. Dressed in sheets and head towels, simulating Universal Precautions, we couldn't stop laughing. We made up rhyming couplets about splashing, splattering, and smearing. It was not a pretty picture.

I WONDERED A lot about whether hospital officials would genuinely listen to the observations of a nursing student, should she make an important discovery, come upon previously unknown information, or observe medical mistakes being made. I never had the opportunity to find out, since I left after my first year of training to get married. (The rules said, "No student will be able to work evenings if she is a married woman.") But that didn't keep me from being curious about the what-ifs.

In the fall of 1953, when I entered Shannon Medical Center's nursing program, my fellow students and I were so immersed in popular culture and societal expectations that we eagerly signed our contracts, promising not to marry until after our graduation. Only one out was offered: we could decide to marry after completing the first year and not be held accountable for room, board, or tuition for that year. I met my obligations to the school during that first year, but I had been proposed to by a handsome air force staff sergeant from New York State, and I decided to take him up on his proposal.

My grades were good, and I completed the initial orientation to floor nursing at Shannon Hospital. It was a fine line I was treading, and I was careful to complete all aspects of that first year before I submitted my resignation from the school.

If I had completed my nursing education in the 1950s, there is a chance that I might have contributed 50 years to the profession. I think I had the potential to be a great nurse. Some of my friends disagree with me; they are convinced that I could never have taken orders willingly enough to have lasted in the nursing field. But why couldn't I have walked the tightrope of marriage and career?

My Mother's Empath

~

Judy Schaefer, RCN, MA

"THE BEST TOOLS you will ever have are your own sound reasoning and your own two hands," a nursing professor told me once, among the noisy beep and click of the ICU. The professor's intelligence and nudging but protective energy were much like my mother's, and they merge together in this poem. Early experiences with my mother taught me an empathy that, although I did not know it at the time, prepared me for a nursing career. I was born during World War II on a farm in Missouri and moved to a small village before the family eventually migrated to Saint Louis. The poem reflects a time of substantial change after the war, from traditional family farming to the "industrialization" of farming.

I. Kindergarten, 1949

The neighbor wipes her mouth
with the hem of her apron,
shouts across the pebbled garden path
from her kitchen door to my mother's porch.

Rain clean and steady on the gray stone,
rain sweet and slow on the kitchen window,
drips and ripples on the pane, imagining . . .
Shot . . . killed his daughter . . .

I push closer into the softness of my mother,
smell flour, apples, and the heated pulse of fear.
Her arm comes around and finds me.
Then . . . killed himself . . .

She nudges—nudges me back, pushes me
into the house, she stretches to hear.
The rain taps. The day suddenly raw.
Cold. Her hair now wet.

Silence—when my brother comes in from school—
whispers—when my father comes in from work.
Candles. Flowers. Perfume.
Prayer worn, wooden pew.

Listening, imagining. Awkward. Listening.
She was pregnant . . . can you imagine . . .
Wax form of a young woman's body in a long box.
Rain clean and steady on the gray stone.

II. School, 1955

The day I became an empath
was the day I became a nurse.
The country hospital smelled of urine
and disinfectant; apple sauce,

powder, rubbing alcohol,
iodine, and graham crackers soaked in milk.
Smells that I feel at home in.
My mother, pale, in a hospital bed

post-op, age thirty-six, temperature rising,
post-op of a total hysterectomy.
My father gone—working, airplane factory.
My brother gone—working, shoe factory.

I, eleven years old, hold her hand
unaware our lives are shifting
no matter how hard we hold on.
Suddenly old, I make adult promises

in response to the heated pulse of her fear.
Do not let them lie to me.
I won't let them lie to you.
In our foothills of the Ozarks

the hospital is where you go to die.
I watch for her, watch her breathe, count, multiply
and divide, coax raindrops to her forehead,
keep influence for her—in case they lie.

III. Flashback, 1947

A farmer with children . . .
He was spared the war . . .
A farmer needs children . . .
We lost the farm, you know.

She dozes, I fall into my own thought:
the summer of the drought,
baby catfish squirm in the pond
digging deep into Missouri mud,

the smell of blood baking.
A dry scar in a fallow field
crusting under high noon sun.
I hear the vibrant scream of fish pain

as only a small child can hear.
I fall down on my knees
in the brown meadow grass.
I place my hands together,

point them to heaven,
pray the first prayer that I really meant.
Remembering—remembering—when my brother
and I saw a long-legged bird,

thought it was a stork and we—we—the first to know
a baby was coming, raced each other home.
While startled at the tumbling waterfall of vivid
        recollection,
I stay put and calmly pray for rain—and she sleeps.

IV. Graduation, Now

A nurse-graduate of childhood
I still lay-me-down-to-sleep, pray-my-soul-to-keep.
I, a witness to pain, an empath, spend my life
on the journey back to the forest, the meadows and
    the fields

where the moss grows
on an ancient stone-circle well
built
horse whisperers
and pioneering ancestors

where brook trout sing
in the splashes of the cool creek
and leap toward mayflies
under blue beads of wild grapes

where long-legged black bugs strut
across the quiet pools
like a memory across a settled thought,
linger there, then quickly scatter.

The lush rain plumps softly
on the summer green canopy.
I push closer into the memory of my mother,
smell flour, apples; recall the pulse of fear.

Her arm comes around and always finds me
teaches me   pushes me

I watch for her, watch her breathe, count each
    respiration
I coax raindrops—now sweet again—to her
    forehead.

Memory Whispers

~

Elizabeth Simpson

"A<small>RE YOU SURE</small> you want to be a nurse?" my father asked in 1959. I was 17 and dreamed of being a modern Florence Nightingale while my parents reminded me that I might be lonely in another city, away from family for the first time.

"How will you manage with strangers?" my mother asked, worried because I had never tended the sick or dying. Nor had I seen a naked person over the age of six. But I had made up my mind. After all, determination was easy for those who grew up in protected families at a time on the Canadian prairies when the mass media were restricted, especially for youth, and the church a central institution in most family life.

At the Regina airport, my 12-year-old sister wept and Grandma give me a dollar to buy a snack. Having come to Canada by boat at the turn of the 20th century, she was unaware that lunch on airplanes was included in the fare. I hugged my family as the prairie wind dusted our eyes and whipped at our clothes. Once on board, I realized that my father, a superstitious man, would have been upset if he saw that my seat bore the unlucky number 13.

I was leaving my home on the Saskatchewan prairies to fly to the Misericordia Hospital in Winnipeg, Manitoba, 400 miles away. A romantic teenager, I had decided to return to the hospital where I had been born, where my grandfather had died when I was 9, and where Mother had undergone surgery when I was 13. Family history had created a path for me in the confines of my limited imagination.

On the plane, I sat beside a woman who told me her son had cut off his hand when he was chopping wood with his father. She wept as she talked about how her boy had changed from a carefree nine-year-old to a child who seldom spoke and hated to go where others could see him. She said her husband had left her because he couldn't live with his guilt and she was now flying to visit her parents because her mother was dying of cancer. I wondered, as she talked, what she had done to anger God. I also fantasized about sewing her son's hand back onto his wrist.

The mother's story and my flights of fancy were interrupted by the stewardess who came to tell me the pilot would like to see me in the cockpit. I wouldn't learn until years later that my father had arranged this opportunity. I simply thought that once a girl began down her chosen path, the world opened up to her. I thought too that once I had my nursing degree, I would be eligible to become a stewardess and save lives when planes crashed or tend to travelers who suffered from motion sickness. My fantasy was interrupted by the two men in uniform who sat behind a canvas curtain and piloted the airplane. They wanted to show me Brandon, Manitoba, the city below that marked the halfway point between Regina and Winnipeg.

"ARE YOU SURE this is the right place?" I asked the taxi driver when he pulled up to a gray building that bore little resemblance to the white hospital on the brochure. I was experiencing my first taxi ride and felt uncomfortable questioning the man behind the wheel. He pointed to the name over the arched door, and I realized the sunny building in the brochure photograph was dimmed by an overcast sky.

Catholic nuns ran the Misericordia Hospital and, although my family was Presbyterian, Mother believed that nuns made the finest nurses and piano teachers. My sister, gifted from birth, played piano with a straight back and clean fingernails as the nuns had taught us, and in the days ahead she would fulfill my parents' dream for her of becoming an accomplished pianist. No one had questioned her chosen career as they did mine.

Eleanor, a graduate nurse, was assigned the role of Big Sister. She led me upstairs to where I stored my clothes in a metal locker and shared a small room with three army cots and two strangers. One of my roommates, Gladys, was as tall as my father and had large eyes magnified by thick glasses. She wore no jewelry, except a man's watch. Delia, my other roommate, was never far from smiles or tears, her dimpled face circled by brown curls.

Twelve girls shared the claw-foot tub and high toilet at the end of the hall. I wedged the rubber bath plug under the door to ensure a moment's privacy in this room without a lock. Someone had left the toilet unflushed, so before I sat down I pulled the dangling chain. A small sign nearby read, "Plugged Do Not Flush." Moments later someone yelled about water leaking from under the bathroom door.

"Weren't you just in there?" Gladys asked. She was 25 and had come from a farming community. Delia was 21, the only child of parents as old as my grandmother. We three went together to our first class, where we learned that germs waited everywhere to cripple the unwashed, encouraging us to use squares of toilet paper to open doors once our hands were scrubbed. I also learned I could not bathe unless I was willing to let other girls come and go as they needed the washroom.

"You'll get the hang of it," Big Sister Eleanor comforted, but she never explained how.

"Lights out!" someone called that night, and a nun's silhouette appeared in our doorway, her hand flicking off the single bulb that hung from the ceiling. "Pull the blind. Men loiter in the street," she said. When she closed our door, I crawled under an itchy gray blanket and woke to a bell to discover morning had already come. Gladys was dressed and sitting in the dark, and soon Delia too was up, her bosom heaving with worry. In the cold bathroom I thought of Mother pouring tea for my grandmother, Father reading his newspaper, and my sister fretting about the seeds in her raspberry jam. I slipped into the chapel to ask God to help me feel less fearful.

Students in the late 1950s went straight onto the wards to work, learning on the job. I pushed patients to and fro in silence, as I exchanged old sheets for fresh ones. When I passed Delia in the hall, I saw the anxiety in her eyes and the spots of red on her cheeks. Gladys was cool and efficient. With long arms she rolled out patients and sheets like cookie dough, not seeming to differentiate between cotton and flesh, male and female, suffering and comfort as she got the job done.

In class we learned that the unmarried girls housed nearby with their swollen bellies deserved our pity. The teacher said some of them tried to use knitting needles to puncture the home of their unborn child. She said death before baptism was a horror far greater than giving birth unwed. No child got to heaven without the priest's blessing. If a nurse had to choose between mother and baby, she must choose the baby. As she spoke, I wondered who would feed the woman's other children and wash their clothes.

When I phoned to ask if I could come home, my mother said discomfort was part of growing up. Father responded to the knitting needles by saying they might be used by pregnant women in big cities, but not by prairie people. I held back my tears and returned to check temperatures, make beds, and glance furtively at the pregnant girls next door.

The first patient I bathed was on the terminal ward. The word *terminal* brought images of platforms where trains came and went. The bed held a 12-year-old girl who was delighted to see me with my bowl of steaming water and my facecloths. "What a big Band-Aid!" I exclaimed, looking at her head as I rolled her onto her side to untie her gown and wash her back.

The girl's voice was as whimsical as a bird's summer song when she said, "The lump behind my ear made me dizzy." In response, I smoothed her sheets and put my palm against her cheek as Mother had done when I was sick. "My dad says I'm as bald as a baby's bum." She laughed before telling me they were from the nearby town of Selkirk and that her father owned a grocery store.

"Mother Gregory doesn't allow us to laugh and talk with patients," Big Sister Eleanor interrupted, referring to the mother superior, the invisible woman who headed the school. Happy chatter would have been wasted on my next patient, an old woman whose body was shrunken like an apple left too long on the kitchen counter. When I moved her, she whimpered, her watery eyes frightened. When I rolled her back, she expelled a stream of liquid moans that tore into my conscience. "You have to do it," Eleanor said.

I picked up the wizened arms that had nothing to cushion the sagging skin that pressed against brittle bone. Humming a lullaby, I uncovered ankles swollen into tissue-paper flesh. "It hurts her," I pleaded.

"No one is too sick for a clean bed," Eleanor told me, grabbing my palm away from the woman's face.

I ran down the hallway, past stretchers lining the walls, and through double doors into the cold and sunny autumn. Blood pounded in my head. One white stocking freed itself from my garter belt and lay bunched around my ankle. When I leaned against a fence to catch my breath, a large golden cat brushed against my leg and I circled its warm body in my arms. When I returned to the lunch room, Delia passed me the remains of her meal, cleaning her cutlery on her apron before handing it to me.

"What did you expect?" Gladys asked, spooning custard into her mouth, one measured spoonful at a time.

I was taken off the terminal ward and put into a ward with people who had broken bones. "It's a man!" I whispered to Eleanor.

"Men break their legs too," she said, telling me he had broken both legs and one arm. "Men are all the same after the first one," she whispered, passing me clean sheets. Even though I kept the sheet over him, I glimpsed a pyramid of white rise as I soaped his thighs. When I complained to Eleanor, she grinned and told me, "It will be gone now." And she was right, but once I lathered anything below the man's chest, the angle of the bedsheet rose again.

Mother Gregory wore a large cross and sat behind a large desk in a dimly lighted room. From within folds of her nun's cap, she said I must not think of patients as men and women, but as God's children. She told me never again to wear my uniform to run about on the streets. She asked me to remember that I had been voted to represent the college in the Freshie Princess competition at the university next month. As she spoke, I was reminded that my mother was laboring over her sewing machine to send a dress for the occasion. "I won't win because I have freckles," I said.

"God marks us in his own way," the mother superior told me, standing up to indicate our talk was over. I waited a moment for her to come around the desk and hug me, but she remained where she was.

I gathered enough coins to phone long-distance and ask about jobs at Eaton's department store in Regina where my parents shopped. The manager said the sock department would need a young woman to help over Christmas, and if my work was satisfactory they might keep me on. With this ammunition, I phoned home to tell my parents that I had a job as a sales clerk in Regina. "Give yourself another month," my father coaxed. "If you're still homesick, I'll send the train fare."

My father's demoting me from airplane to train seemed a mild rebuke in comparison to Mother's saying, "I will not abide a quitter." My father had been orphaned young, and compassion came readily to him. I heard my mother's heels click on the linoleum as she walked away, my father calling after her to say he would allow me two weeks to rest up at home.

Years would pass before I took my parents to the Faculty Club at the University of British Columbia and proved to them I could succeed at something as long as it required teaching literature instead of tending wounded bodies. Still later, in middle age, I would suffer a serious cancer that reminded me of those angels of mercy who toughed it out to tend those as sick and helpless as myself.

But back in 1959 it seemed the evening train took forever to arrive on the windy autumn platform in Winnipeg. An hour before midnight, white smoke poured from the engine and I climbed aboard. The unspeakable grief of failure traveled with me as the lights of prairie towns and the dusky images of grain elevators rose against an expanse of darkness. When dawn spread across the prairies, I hadn't slept. November frost had petrified the remnants of harvest as snow dusted the farmlands. I had no idea where Manitoba ended and Saskatchewan began, but an hour before noon the landscape opened onto the familiar outskirts of Regina.

"Dad!" I called as I stepped from the train and ran toward my father's green and smiling eyes, our frosty breath mingling as we hugged. Grandma was waiting with him, warm inside her ankle-length muskrat coat. She seemed an aged version of myself, a woman who had come to live with my parents when she was widowed and had nowhere else she wanted to be. I realized now what it had meant when she had lost Grandpa to his illness years before. Who, I wondered, would ease the terrible and precious moments in the lives of the elderly and dying if nurses refused their duties as I had done?

"She will return after Christmas," my mother said to my father, as though I weren't sitting with them at the table. "Otherwise she will bring shame to our family."

"We'll give her two weeks," my father told her. "She needs time to think things through."

Without my realizing it at the moment, my father's word set a new path for me, one that required I think things through before I ventured off again, that I examine my aptitudes before I dreamed my way into another disaster. Perhaps more powerful was my hope that I would never again bring shame to my mother or put my father in a position of having to defend me. I would pay him back for his faith in me and I would prove to my mother that a daughter can think things through as she sells socks in Eaton's and then sets out again on a path that allows her to cultivate her strengths.

Sisters of Charity

~

Nina Howes, RN

AFTER HER STROKE, at the Sisters of Charity nursing home, Grandmother spoke in long sentences that didn't make sense, called me *Rosa, Gloria, Nellie.* I sat near her and nodded, watching the Sisters work, pulling the curtain around the patients' beds. Their white-stockinged legs moved from one bed to another. When they were finished, a freshly bathed patient appeared from behind the curtain, sitting up, a fluffed pillow behind her, a smooth white sheet folded neatly across her chest. The Sisters moved on to the next bed, doing the same amazing dance.

I Am a Real Nurse

~

Cheryl Herndon, MSN, CNM, ARNP

"I AM JUST AN LPN," responds the young nurse to my inquiry regarding her job. She leans forward and gently wipes the drool from my aging mother's lips.

A few days later, I report to an outpatient facility for my yearly blood profile. "I'm just a lab nurse," apologizes the RN who draws my blood.

Something about the word *just* grates on me like fingernails screeching on an old-fashioned blackboard, and the phrase *just a,* in reference to any profession, and especially to nursing, is one I would love to see eliminated from the English language.

As for me, I am a certified nurse-midwife and an advanced registered nurse practitioner. It has been my experience that many nurses make "just a" statements when I reveal my advanced credentials. My immediate response to such a statement is "There is no such thing as a just a _____."

If I am not a "just a," what am I? I consider myself first and foremost a real nurse. When I think of the initials *RN* after my name, I affirm in my own mind that I am a real nurse as well as a registered nurse. I chose to further my education by obtaining my master's degree, and I chose to specialize in women's healthcare, but I am first a real nurse. If only to amuse my own ego, I often introduce myself with the greeting "Hi, my name is Cheryl, and I am a real nurse."

Nursing to me is more than a career. It's part of my identity. Nursing is my calling, a purpose and a venue for giving back to others. To me, these qualities define a real nurse.

My personal career path as a nurse has changed over the past 20 years. I remember that when I decided to go to nursing school, one of my first instructors explained that a nurse is more than a bedpan changer or medication dispenser. She emphasized that a nurse is also an educator, a motivator, a researcher, and a role model. This concept broadened my perception of the nursing role. I also remember being shocked a few weeks into nursing school to discover many, if not most, of my fellow nursing students had not entered the profession to help other people. They did not necessarily consider nursing a calling or an avenue through which to give back to others. They wanted to be nurses to ensure job security and flexible schedules. Some of my fellow nursing students actually admitted that they didn't even like people! Have you ever met *that* nurse?!

Nursing started out for me as a means to an end. Initially, I simply wanted to deliver babies. In the early 1970s, the legal way to attend births was to become a physician or midwife.

At that time I was not so much interested in being a nurse as I was in becoming a birth attendant. Early on, I realized that in order to have any significant influence, I would need credibility. My initial educational journey was frustrating because few institutions of higher learning offered nurse-midwifery as a degree program.

When I began taking nursing prerequisite courses, there were no RN programs within 100 miles of where I lived. By the time I was ready for nursing school, a bachelor of science in nursing (BSN) program became available within commuting distance.

I now believe that being educated first as a nurse was the best foundation I could have for reaching my personal goals. Nursing fundamentals are life values that are applicable in almost every arena. I am so thankful to have been encouraged and mentored by a few exceptional "real nurses" who encouraged me in pursuing my own dreams. Dedicated nurses motivated me to forge ahead.

One nurse wisely told me, "Don't worry whether or not specific doors will open for you in the future. Let today's worries be sufficient for this day."

My nurse friend went on to say, "Nursing is the epitome of flexibility. Trust your future to the future." She was right. By the time I arrived at a juncture where I was ready to take the next step, the right doors did open for me.

Upon completing my BSN, I worked for two years as a labor and delivery nurse. I learned to truly appreciate various positions nurses fulfilled in a hospital setting. I did not particularly like floor nursing. It was often physically exhausting. Worse, I usually felt powerless in decision making. I longed for autonomy and the ability to make my own management decisions in patient care.

Most nursing programs recommend an obligatory two years working as a medical-surgical nurse immediately after graduation from nursing school. I never did the recommended rotation as a med/surgical nurse and still don't regret the decision. My heart was always in maternal/child healthcare. I did not want to take care of acutely sick people or even take care of men, for that matter. I wanted to focus on wellness care for women, health maintenance issues, and overall support of pregnant women, which was something I felt nurse-midwifery encompassed.

Upon completing my two years as a labor and delivery nurse, I began my search for a quality master's program. I was accepted and graduated from the University of Illinois at Chicago. Here, I again realized that, just as an RN can specialize, so can a nurse-midwife. Opportunities varied from teaching nursing at a college, to working in infertility management, to delivering babies in birth centers. The choices seemed unlimited.

My first job as a midwife was in a freestanding birthing center. I worked there for a few years assisting with low-risk deliveries in a beautiful, safe, homelike setting. This nursing role provided a great deal of autonomy and responsibility. I grew to appreciate and depend on other nurses who worked with me. That nurse/nurse-midwife team was incredibly cohesive and powerful in providing quality care for women.

I continued as a nurse-midwife working in both hospitals and clinics for more than 15 years. I had reached my goal to be a real nurse. One of the problems with my success is that I became too busy. Being a good nurse or nurse-midwife puts one in great demand. I worked too many hours for too long until, at age 52, personal health problems forced me to change my lifestyle.

Lying on my back incapacitated, staring at little holes in the ceiling tile, provided me with an unexpected midlife opportunity for self-evaluation.

What next? I pondered. I was a nurse. I was a nurse-midwife, and a very good one at that. But during my period of convalescence, I began to embrace that "just a" feeling. I wondered if I was still a real nurse or "just a nurse."

It was during this time of contemplation I thought through the character qualities of a nurse. The simple principles I learned in Nursing 101 of the nursing process were still solid guidelines. The principles work. Whether or not I had the title of RN or a salary that reflected a career in nursing did not negate the fact that I am a real nurse. I realized that helping can occur daily, even from a supine bedridden state. Self-improvement can continue until a person draws her last breath. Nursing is relational. I realized I wanted to continue working with people and being a nurse.

I experienced a complete career change. I am still in nursing. I am still working primarily with women, but now I am working as a nurse-practitioner providing cosmetic laser services. The years I spent petitioning for the right of women to be spared from having their pubic hair shaved during childbirth have been replaced by years of removing that same "sacred" hair permanently with laser. I have to laugh at the irony. Nursing means helping the patient obtain what she wants, not want I think she wants. I am still a real nurse taking care of real women.

My current role as a nurse who provides cosmetic laser services is not only easy and stress free but also has regular defined hours with no nights and weekends (the nurse's dream)! My personal health is now completely restored. I am enjoying this current phase of my life.

However, when I encounter former coworkers, I occasionally catch myself saying, "I am just a laser nurse now." I suddenly realize what I have inadvertently confessed and quickly correct myself. I am still a nurse. I am relating to women. I assess, plan, implement, and evaluate every single person I care for. I encourage, educate, and empower the women who come to me for their laser care. I listen to others more than I ever did earlier in my career. Perhaps now I truly represent nursing. I am an RN. I am a nurse-midwife. The definition of *midwife* is "with woman." As a nurse-midwife, I stand beside women in their life journey, in the truest sense. I am not just a nurse. I am a *real* nurse.

I Will *Not* Be a Schoolteacher!

~

Royce Jane Uyechi, RN, BSN

AT EVERY FAMILY get-together, I listened to my schoolteacher mother and her five schoolteacher sisters discussing school issues. Their conversations revolved around bulletin boards, lesson plans, difficult students, and problem parents. I was determined that I would not follow family tradition. I would follow my own career path and it would definitely *not* be teaching.

But what would it be? How about nursing? Hmmmm, that seemed like a good possibility, so I began my research into what being a nurse involved.

My father's sister, Aunt Irene, was an RN. I looked at her in admiration when I saw her in her immaculate white starched uniform, her white stockings and sensible white oxfords, and her crown of a stiff white cap. She was efficient, always calm, and ever kind and gentle. She unknowingly helped me become fascinated with the mysteries of nursing. Her nursing textbooks in my grandmother's attic became my own private treasure trove when I went to visit. I eagerly devoured all of the books with their strange and secret words and pictures, especially the anatomy ones.

My senior year in high school, I had an opportunity to work side by side with a real RN. As a clinic aide, I watched the school nurse care for students every day. I have a clear picture of her with her crisp white blouses, navy blue skirts, black oxfords, short salt-and-pepper hair, and wide smile. She was calm and efficient as she skillfully handled all of the varied situations that confronted her as a school nurse. There were tearful conferences with students behind her private office door, hasty trips to other parts of the school carrying her black bag, and stacks of paperwork to be done. She became my shining example to follow in my later years as a school nurse.

In the fall of 1961, I began my quest for the coveted white cap at Texas Woman's University College of Nursing. Campus life was great fun, and the courses were challenging. The very first semester of my freshman year, Nursing 101: The History of Nursing was my beginning step into the field of nursing. The second semester brought Nursing 102: The Fundamentals of Nursing, in which we began to practice "real nursing" on each other—taking temperatures and blood pressures, transferring patients, offering bedpans, and giving bed baths. Bed baths! Here my idealized picture of being a wonderful nurse whom everyone adored came crashing down around me. I made the horrifying discovery that I did not like touching other people's bodies. But I still loved nursing—and I was *not* going to be a schoolteacher.

I reconciled that discrepancy between the ideal and the real by discovering what I really had a heart for: teaching nursing. Clinical rotations became a necessary evil, something that I had to grit my teeth and endure in order to get that black velvet band around my white cap. And I knew that I couldn't teach something that I had not learned myself. With this new goal in mind, I began to observe my instructors more closely, to learn not just what they were teaching but also how they were teaching it. What methods excited me to dig deeper into the subject? What projects fueled my imagination to create a better way of doing things? What made lectures exciting and what made them deadly boring? What personal interactions inspired me to become an excellent nurse rather than just an adequate one?

My instructor for the senior comprehensive nursing course was a teacher of the make-you-or-break-you mold and an awe-inspiring icon of TWU. I trembled each time she walked onto the unit. She looked around, taking in everything, and seemed to see straight into my soul before she began asking her infamous question: "Why?" If my response was uncertain or unsubstantiated, she looked at me skeptically and left me with an admonition: "Look it up." Many times I was chagrined to discover that I had given her the correct answer but had failed to defend that answer with confidence. I emerged from her tutelage with a confidence in myself as a nurse that launched me out into the real world with a sure step.

I graduated and earned the white uniform, the white shoes and stockings, and the cap with a black velvet stripe that identified me as a registered nurse. After a year of staff nursing, I entered my true calling: teaching nursing. I loved it and found irony in my pleasure at preparing lesson plans, motivating indifferent students, and even conferencing with the difficult parent who challenged me in the dean's office about the failing grade that her daughter earned in my class.

Marriage and motherhood brought years of varied part-time work until I returned to full-time nursing—as a school nurse. All of those hours of listening to teacher stories had given me a unique perspective to bring to this job. I understood teachers' desire to have students leave a class with more knowledge than they came in with, and their frustration with anything that interfered with that goal. Requests from the school nurse definitely fell into that category. They saw my job as getting students back to the classroom as soon as possible or sending them home quietly so that they didn't spread their germs. I learned to find the least obtrusive times to call students in for screenings or admonitions about getting their immunizations. Most important, I found ways to teach. Every student who walked into my clinic represented a golden teaching opportunity: "Your ankle is swollen because . . ." "The best way to treat that sunburn is . . ." "It is time to go see a doctor about this when . . ." "You must take every single antibiotic because . . ." "The steps to getting rid of these head lice are . . ."

After 20 rewarding years, I retired from the public schools. But I was not ready to retire completely. The question was "What should I do?" I considered some options:

(1) Hospital nursing was a possibility, but my 60-year-old body wouldn't be able to hold up to the pace, my clinical skills were way beyond rusty, and I had never liked hospital nursing anyway. (2) Health education in a nonprofit organization was appealing, but positions were scarce, work might be erratic, and jobs usually depended on grant money, which could be unreliable. (3) Working outside the nursing profession would be fun, but my years of nursing experience would be wasted, I might have to have additional schooling, and the pay could be minimal.

Then I discovered health coaching and found my perfect match. This emerging field of nursing requires all of the skills that are my strengths: teaching and encouraging people, engaging them in interactions, finding creative solutions, and talking on the telephone all day. As a health coach, I have the opportunity to make a meaningful impact on the health of many people. Through educating them, I empower them to be active participants in their own healthcare, help them to manage their chronic conditions, and guide them in making healthy lifestyle choices. As I make follow-up calls and establish relationships, I get immediate feedback on how I have had a positive effect on people's lives. I know that what I am doing is making a difference to change America's health, one person at a time.

Wouldn't all my schoolteacher aunts be surprised to see me now? Here I am, doing what I vowed I would *not* do—teaching! And loving it!

Homeostasis

~

Kelly Sievers, CRNA

Arching ureters curved from bladder to kidneys,
    filling the blackboard.
Tubules twined to Loops of Henle, while
    buffers calmed acids,
salt scuttled in and out. We squinted

into the alchemy. Miss Huegelon said,
    "Ho-me-o-sta-sis
is beautiful." She said it so many times
    Patty began to kick me.
I looped the world with tight circles, watched

Ginny twirl a loose lock beneath her cap
    around and over, around
and over. Alerted mothers had sent us here.
    They saw a speeding wheel

of war, a shattering of paradigms.
    Nursing would spare us.

Miss Huegelon stood erect, her blue-gray hair
    jiggled in tiny knobs,
brown serge dipped to her oxfords. She spoke
    slowly while we counted
waves of purple veins along her temple,
    felt her terror.

Grannie, the
Would-Be Nurse

~

Ann Neuser Lederer, RN, BSN

GRANNIE ALWAYS WANTED to become a nurse. She
was born in 1896, and her mother maintained old-fashioned
ideas about acceptable behavior for young ladies. In those
days, nursing carried a taint of the unrespectable. Grannie's
mother was born in Canada in 1862, of parents who had
escaped the poverty of Ireland. Nursing duties in that era
included mopping and cooking, resembling perhaps too
much the work of maids, likely an unpleasant stereotype to
be avoided for a daughter of Irish immigrants. Before mar-
rying, Grannie's mother had worked as a milliner, surely
an occupation more elegant than cleaning up the messes of
the infirm.

Grannie was only nine years old when her father died.
She and her three sisters, their father's "little princesses,"

along with their mother moved hundreds of miles north to a city where Grannie's uncle lived. He could help look after the fatherless family. Because her mother disapproved of her desire to become a nurse, Grannie compromised and, after graduating from high school in 1914 (just before the outbreak of World War I), went on to normal school to study to become a dietitian. With her dietitian's diploma, Grannie moved to Chicago at the age of 20 to take a hospital job there. She also became active in the women's suffrage movement. Before the end of the war, she moved back to her mother's town and continued to practice as a dietitian in a local hospital.

The 1918 flu epidemic caused staffing shortages and overwhelming workloads, so Grannie pitched in to assist the doctors and nurses with tasks such as answering phones and collecting names and addresses of patients flooding into the hospital. In 1919, Grannie married and soon had three daughters of her own. She was no longer employed in hospitals. But many years later she started volunteering in one, where she worked for years. Wearing her peach-colored volunteer's smock and her trademark gracious smile, she delighted in staffing the information desk or carrying greeting cards to patients in their rooms. At age 90, frail with illness, she finally handed in her resignation, but the director of volunteers said instead that her name would be put on the "leave of absence" list. This thought pleased Grannie. She never officially quit working in that hospital. It was the hospital of my birth.

As a girl, I did not aspire to become a nurse, but I remember hearing often about Grannie's thwarted plans.

After studying anthropology in college, and then being hit with the reality of a tight job market, I accepted work in a nursing home as an aide. A whole new world opened to my eyes. Most of the residents there had been born in Europe, and many were refugees from Hitler. I was assigned to the back ward, home of the oldest, the most ill, the most demented, and the most needy. I surprised myself by falling in love there with the people and the work. Although bone-tired at the end of each shift, I began to imagine myself as a nurse. I mentioned this idea to Grannie, who was thrilled. Some of the nurses at the facility, mostly older women and well seasoned, gave me advice. Don't get so attached, they warned. But they also provided unforgettable examples of competent, loving care in the face of difficult challenges, and encouraged me to apply to nursing school.

Before long, I was attending an associate degree nursing (ADN) program at a local community college, and continued to work part-time, first in that nursing home and later as a ward clerk in a psychiatric hospital. My nursing school encouraged students to take the LPN exam after their first year of classes, and after passing, I went back to work part-time at my original nursing home, this time as a nurse. I passed meds and charted, suddenly feeling very professional. I was also getting useful experience for my remaining training as an RN.

By this time, Grannie was already using the phrase "my granddaughter, the nurse" to describe me, making me feel official and proud. Eventually, at my first hospital job, I had the privilege of caring for a 101-year-old blind man. Born in the South, he had polite manners that echoed the old days.

He always greeted me and the other nurses as "Sister," a now nearly archaic honorific. Somehow, this title caused my mind to reverberate back to Grannie and her times, maybe because the nurse's training from her day was often convent based, including street women who had nowhere else to turn. Although I have now been in nursing for more than 25 years, to this day when I hear someone call out "Nurse," I feel in some way that I am fulfilling at least a tiny part of Grannie's ongoing dream.

She Wants
to Be a Nurse

~

Andrea Vlahakis, RN

3–11 shift.
One of *those* nights. If it can go wrong,
    it does.
Too many patients.
Never enough of us.
Rushing back to the nurse's station, I'm stopped
    by a patient's husband.
Standing behind him—barely waist high—
    his granddaughter.
She is shy, but her eyes are lit, eager, like
    a racehorse at the gate.
"She wants to be a nurse," he says.
I stop.
And kneel down.

I recognize something in her face. I know
    she will be filling my shoes
    when the time comes. And that time will come.
She touches my stethoscope with fingers gentle
    and unafraid.
I place the earpieces in her ears and let her
    hear her heart beat.
Listen, I tell her. *All the patients you will ever
    care for are there — in those heartbeats —
    waiting for you.* But
she already knows this.

On Becoming a Nurse

~

Juliette Ast Dols, RN

So you jump. You tell yourself, *I want something different, something more. I want to do and be more.* And you jump. You don't know where your feet will land, how the terrain will look, what passersby will say or do or want. You know that you are following this urge inside you; you believe it comes from your soul, God nudging you on your way. Different people call it different things. To you, it's something you can't ignore, so you listen. You quit your job, you go into debt, you hang up your dress pants and shirts, you put aside your travels, and you say good-bye to what you know. And then you land . . . where? I'm still not sure. . . .

Suddenly you enter a culture of authority, of rigidity, of ways of doing things that are decades old. Many of your future work colleagues are your mother's or your grandmother's age. Even the "young" have been in the field for 20 years. They're tired, hardened, and burned out, and they ask you why of all careers you chose this one. For a few moments, maybe more, you ask yourself the same thing. You walk down halls where people don't speak to each other, where titles can mean everything, where patients become subjects. You spend hours with a patient and wonder if those who write the orders even listen or read your input; you know they don't acknowledge you when they enter the patient's room. You watch physicians and nurses, all clinicians, dance around a patient: they pour out their own opinions, they do their job as they were taught—they write orders, they take orders, they chart and chart and chart. And the patient lies there questioning, *What is this dance?* As on a doomed all-star team, the players focus on their own fame, on their own winning moves, and they forget to play as a team. Perhaps it's ego, fear, ignorance, or just "the way it's always been." But in the center is a person who relies on you, hopeful that these people will get together enough so that he or she can return home without complications.

You leave the hospital and go to school. You know your teachers mean well. They want bright, competent nurses—clinicians that will help save lives. Many are supportive, encouraging, inspiring. There are others who seem to believe, as they were likely taught, that they have to break you down to see what you're worth, to make you tough; you just hope they don't break you into too many small pieces. For a minute you wonder, *Why am I here?*

And then you take a moment and breathe. You take in all that you've given up, that you've learned, that you've gained. You remind yourself that, if you were looking for a picnic, you should have selected a field where daily headlines don't mention crises: the nursing shortage, the increasing costs and decreasing resources, the increasing demands and decreasing patient satisfaction, the underserved, the uninsured—the list could go on and on. If you wanted to believe that life is always sweet and rosy, maybe you should have avoided caring for a 13-year-old boy brain-dead from cardiac arrest, or carrying a stillborn baby to a grieving mother so she could seek closure from her loss.

You finally get honest, you take a deep breath, and you transcend. You return to that urge inside of you and you remind yourself that if you truly want to fuel change, you go where the need is greatest. You know you've been accused of being idealistic. You've been told you'll burn out too, just like the rest. You know you've already felt the pang of doubt and wonder how strong that doubt can get. You feel yourself getting tired as you try not to succumb to the status quo that surrounds you. You remind yourself that you haven't even gotten to where you want to go: you have more years of school, more uncertainties, more responsibility. You know that your vision looks different from how things currently are, and you wonder if you've really got what it takes to actually change things—anything, however small. You have no idea what lies ahead of you, what surprises exist, but you believe and you hope that things can be different.

You continue to listen to that urge inside you; you look to your soul, to God. You smile as you think about where you've been and what you've learned. You recognize what gives you strength, and you begin to hoard it. You're going to need it. You start to find humor in this backward culture. You begin to see peace in loss. You start to recognize hope in sickness, in death. You begin to rebuild your confidence and feel good about what you do, about who you are and what you are becoming. . . .

So you jumped. You pick yourself up and regain your balance. You look around and realize that what you see is Life, true Life. You could have stayed in a safe place where everyone looks and acts the same, where people go away when ill and return when well. But you decide to see Life exposed. You realize that Life is people. It's you and the stranger next to you. It's both beautiful and ugly. It's chaos. It's order. It's happiness, sadness, love, and suffering. Life is egos and greed. Life is selflessness. Life is sickness. Life is miracles. . . .

You jumped. You pick yourself up. You laugh. You cry. You live.

PART TWO

The Reckoning

Reservations endemic to
the clash of idealism

Winter Count

~

Veneta Masson, RN, MA

Among several tribes on the northern plains,
the passage of time from one summer to the
next was marked noting a single memorable event.
The sequence of such memories . . .
was called a winter count.

—Barry Lopez

1958   Future Nurses Club, junior high. We are photo-
graphed outside the clinic cottage wearing white caps.
Becoming a nurse has somehow occurred to me.

1959   YMCA medical seminar. We tour the coroner's
office in Los Angeles. I see naked bodies in long
rows, think of the frogs we dissected in biology lab.

1960   Junior volunteer. I push the water cart. A patient's
call light blips on. I am terrified of what may be
asked of me. Patient asks for water.

1961   In my senior yearbook, Mr. Olson writes, "Doctor! I'll expect to hear of your accomplishments." Becoming a doctor has never occurred to me.

1962   The two comatose ladies in room 360. I am the nursing student assigned to them each clinical day. I learn to talk to them but do not wonder about their lives.

1963   I am immobilizing a post-op cataract patient with sandbags. Someone whispers that the president has been shot. I retreat to the linen closet.

1964   Dr. P. yells at me in the hallway. His wife is dying. She is our patient. I am the RN in charge. I do not know how to respond.

1965   ER. Summer of the Watts riots. We attempt to resuscitate an old woman whose skull was crushed in a car crash. The doctor won't give up. Why?

1966   Back in school. I buy a paperback poetry collection to read on the bus while commuting to class, discover a poem called "Strokes."

1967   Visiting nurse. Walter is paraplegic, lewd, incorrigible. Lives alone above a bar. Roaches flit across his calendar girl's face, my shoes. I bathe him, fend him off.

1968   My stroke patient Mrs. J. says if there's something in life you want to do, do it now. She says she and her husband waited too long. I go to Europe.

1969   Summer job. I am sent to cover the ICU over dinner break. First time in ICU. I feed a patient dinner. We talk. I like him. He dies. I am compelled to write about this.

1970   Grad school. We read Kafka's "Metamorphosis" in a nursing theory course. I find it bracing, baffling. Patients don't turn into insects. Do they?

1971   My story about the death in the ICU wins me a trip to the Bread Loaf Writers' Conference in Vermont, where I learn that it is a bad story.

1972   I apply to work in international health. I want to go to Africa but am sent to Laredo, Texas. Still, it is *la frontera.*

1973   Brazil, hospital ship. Brazilian nurses work as counterparts to Americans and bunk deep in the bowels of the ship. I have a private cabin and a porthole.

1974   Brazil, the new hospital. We have no water. Doctors protest poor facilities by refusing to see patients and sitting in their cars outside in the parking lot.

1975   I meet Frank over *cafezinho* at the Brazilian-American Cultural Institute in Washington, D.C. We live in the same neighborhood, study Portuguese, marry.

1976   Guatemalan Highlands, after the earthquake. Cold in June. I am jolted out of bed in the middle of the night. Nurses are needed here but, above all, endurance.

1977   Morocco. Government officials want state-of-the-art ICUs. One tells me he admires the American nurse. She is like the captain of a ship.

1978   Washington, D.C. Community Medical Care opens its doors. I am cofounder with Jim. We offer primary care and home care. It is in a poor neighborhood.

1979   Christopher and Emma come for prenatal care. They have no insurance. Emma speaks no English. When Maria Carmen is born, I am asked to be godmother.

1980   I compare my work as a nurse with Jim's as a physician. He wears a lab coat. I do not. He narrows his focus. I do not. I write these observations in a journal.

1981   My book on international nursing is published. It is bright orange with no cover art. I am pleased with the book but not its cover. A chapter of my life closes.

1982   Lease expires. We move in January. Pipes freeze in new clinic. Jim and I have a falling out. He drives me home, wonders how we can continue to work together.

1983   Jim and I teach a course called Healing the Whole Person. One session is on healing relationships. There are two on forgiveness.

1984   L.J. sits naked in her crowded apartment after the stroke. Tells me not to worry about money, a dollar a day is what she'll pay for home care.

1985   Maggie's old mutt traps me on the stairway as I try
       to leave her house. I have fed it, fed her. I am fed
       up. With strokes of my pen, I turn my anger into
       a poem.

1986   Margaret nods off on the toilet seat in the clinic's
       only bathroom. All morning, patients and staff exer-
       cise continence. Margaret is a very mean drunk.

1987   I tell L.M. that his HIV test has come back posi-
       tive. He is our first positive. He is shaken. I learn to
       deliver bad news.

1988   I write columns for a nursing journal about life in
       the clinic and healthcare in the United States. I write
       about money, AIDS, doctors' work, nurses' work.

1989   I study medicine and pharmacology at the university.
       It is both more and less complicated than the care of
       real patients. I am certified as a nurse-practitioner.

1990   I have surgery. My uterus is detached. I detach. I
       enjoy sweet, slow days on the front porch. My patient,
       Ms. Mary, stumps up the front steps bearing cakes.

1991   I sit at the feet of Our Lady, Queen of Ireland, in
       the shrine. Baby Jesus is on her lap. My Salvadoran
       patients grieve for the children they have left
       behind.

1992   Outward Bound. Rock climbing above the Rio
       Grande. I can't climb back up the way I came down.
       I learn to look for another place on the rock.

1993   I try working evenings in urgent care at the HMO. Dr. O. greets me cheerfully, says she works well with "mid-levels." No footholds on this part of the rock.

1994   I wait with Rebecca in the pre-op hold area. R. is my sister. She has breast cancer. The room is cold. Needle caps and spent bandages litter the floor.

1995   Lease expires. The clinic renews. I do not. Jim gives me the pinecone he brought back from the retreat we led at Big Bear in California.

1996   Women's clinic. After examining L., I slide my notebook out of the desk drawer, write, "The hush that falls as my fingers hesitate over the left breast . . ."

1997   Jack and I drive Rebecca home after last-ditch treatment in Mexico. She is comatose. We get stuck at the border. Buy piñatas for the children.

1998   I leave the women's clinic for a study tour of traditional healing in Navajo country. I do not return to it. I will use my hands to write and to bless.

Supreme Love
and Caring

~

Colleen O'Brien, RN, BSN

I AM A MUSICIAN and a nurse. I love to play music and sing. I don't love being a nurse, though I like it and have learned almost everything about people, life, death, and relationships through my experience as a nurse.

I think the seeds were planted fairly early for me to become a nurse. My mom came home from the hospital with her gallstone in a baby jar when I was about 11 years old. She had a huge gallstone, about the size of a large marble. I became fascinated with all things medically related—illness, disease, surgery, the body. In fact, at night I would read from *The Reader's Digest Family Health Guide and Medical Encyclopedia,* and kept it next to my bed, like a Bible.

My mother had many conditions that I could read about. High blood pressure, kidney problems, headaches. Later, when I was a young nurse, she had breast cancer, heart problems, then lymphoma, but what really did her in was her chemotherapy.

I gradually became less enchanted with nursing. At one point I felt so ill about going to see my patients, many of whom I had followed and had taken care of for years, that I needed a break. When my son was three years old, he, my husband, and I packed away all of our things and headed out on an adventure to Alaska. We ended up in the Shangri-la of the north, Homer, Alaska.

Don't get me wrong—I loved my patients. But I needed time with my family in a new environment, doing something different. This particular year was the beginning of my healing, away from nursing.

We found a charming cabin that came with a dog, a cat, and children's books. The cabin overlooked Cook Inlet and the volcanoes of the Alaska Range in the distance. We had an outhouse with a Styrofoam seat and no door, thus the marvelous view of the mountains. We could also see the northern lights at night, all with a warm behind. This was heaven to me. We were a very happy family!

I met my husband while playing music; I hired him for a new band that I was putting together. He was the most musical drummer I had ever heard. During our time in Alaska, we developed a new musical combination of instruments with voice, vibraphone, and cello that turned out to be one of my most favorite combinations of instruments and sounds to this day. We played music every day, and soon we were playing often for the folks of Homer, Alaska. We were so excited by this new instrumentation and music that we moved to the San Francisco Bay area to try our luck with our newfound sound. It soon became clear that we were not meant for the commercial venues: I started feeling that ill feeling again. After I let go of the idea making a living as a commercial musician, the music continued to evolve and has become a life source, a treasure, a sublime sanity in this world that lately has seemed so insane. It is a place of supreme love and caring for connection of heart, mind, and soul and for connection with others.

There were moments caring for patients that I felt like this, but the systems of healthcare, the demand on nurses, the time constraints, the charting, the rules, and the business aspect of medicine all gradually took their toll. Now my feelings about nursing can be compared to having post-traumatic stress disorder. Recently I was listening to an American soldier describe his feelings after having gone to Iraq a couple of times, and it sounded close to how I feel whenever I think about doing hands-on nursing again.

My relationship with nursing is rooted in my childhood, in idealism, in thinking I could help alleviate suffering but discovering my own suffering in the process. I still care for people, but I no longer need to take care of people. I will take care of people if they need me, but I don't think I will be a "commercial" nurse again.

So what about the music? I've always come back to the music. My mother made sure that I could play and sing, and she was my main support. Now that I have my own music, it is inside of me and is a part of my life. Nursing is also a part of my life, in the knowledge gained from years of caring for people. Nursing allowed me to help my mother die; my music has allowed me to live.

Loaded

~

Jenna Rindo, RN

A range of opaque white
covers the still green night nurse.
It's summer in Tallahassee, and the heft
of support hose has her sweating behind both knees.
She ran over a possum on her way to work that night.
The double thud of front and back tires left her
disturbed and doubting her visual memory.
She called home right after shift report,
convinced her husband to leave cotton sheets and
    the oscillating fan
to locate and identify her unavoidable roadkill.

She slides open the glass doors on her most critical
    patient first,
convinces his mom to change into scrubs in lieu
    of pajamas

while she charts his vitals and hangs
miniature bags of antibiotics,
their chartreuse colors welcoming as a neon
    vacancy sign
yet caustic as sweet-tasting antifreeze.
It seems the gun was in the glove box of his
    grandpa's truck.
The obligatory pickup truck with or without
a Confederate flag draped in the rear cab window.
The naive nurse maintains sterile fields with fences
    and drapes,
listens intently for bowel sounds around abdominal
    dressings
but finds all four quadrants ominously quiet.
His young blood leaves a batik on her chart.

During the morning drive home she turns the radio up.
NPR reports the haggling over concealed-weapon laws
while she still smells the nine-year-old boy's
gut gone septic.

Lifting Up

~

Teresa Kenas, RN

WHEN I WAS four years old, my mom and dad took me to a game farm petting zoo where children could feed the smaller animals with baby bottles provided by an attendant. Adorable baby goats gathered around me, just a few at first. They were my size, and we stood eye to eye. Then more goats quickly approached from all directions, their target the one nipple on the bottle in my small hand. Within seconds I became overwhelmed and began sobbing, too young to articulate that fear was not the cause of my dismay. I cried because I couldn't feed them all. I just couldn't! I simply didn't have enough. There was one nipple, room for only one goat, yet they surrounded me, pushing and shoving, almost toppling me over, nearly smothering me with their need.

By nature, I am exquisitely sensitive. My compassion runs deep. My empathy can be excruciating. It's a safe bet that most people do not recognize this depth of emotion in me because of psychological barriers I have constructed over the years. In fact, at times I may even appear indifferent. The opposite is true.

The nursing profession consists of a widespread array of individuals who bring myriad talents and abilities to their work. Among these individuals are my mother, my sister, and my two cousins. So it was to nursing that I brought my own sensibilities and good intentions 26 years ago, when team nursing was de rigueur, when HMOs and managed care were ideas flickering in the distance.

Reality shock waves hit hard my first year. Staffing was short, and we nurses often went to work when we felt ill ourselves, running to get routine tasks completed, finally having time to take a bathroom break, inhaling food during a 10-minute lunch because the long line in the cafeteria devoured the other precious 20 minutes.

I admit that I did not have the tools early on to care for myself in a way that replenished and restored the emotional energy I gave in my work, but it took me a few years to realize the extent of it.

On one particularly awful winter day in New York, every RN on the ear, nose, and throat unit had called in sick. This left me the only RN available to take charge on a unit unfamiliar to me. It never occurred to me to say no. A regular day might not have been so bad, but we were filled above capacity with patient beds in the solarium. Charts flagged with new doctor's orders were stacked ten high and climbing as post-op patients returned from the recovery room. At three o'clock, one patient coded.

When I finally looked outside, I saw that it had been snowing. After giving report to the next shift, I walked down the hall to the pay phone and called the Traveling Nurse Corps. I thought at least a change in weather would do me good.

Travel nursing actually kept nursing itself a viable professional option for me. I joined Flying Nurses and other agencies, and no longer committed to one institution. The opportunity to provide supplemental staffing nationwide was not only about having fun but also about staying sane. Indulging in my love of travel while getting to know new places, new people, and even new customs was enough to distract me from the truth that simmered beneath the surface. I had the training, the compassion, and the work ethic it takes to be a nurse. I did not have the emotional tools to survive as one.

Travel nursing bought me time, but eight years later the nursing shortage was as big a problem as ever. It was a beautiful sunny California day when I was assigned to be team leader for 30 patients. I had only one nurse's aide to help me. Legally, she could not perform any of the multiple treatments necessary, but she answered call bells and helped with vital signs and admissions. Three patients were transferring to my wing, while one was going bad quickly, necessitating transfer to the ICU.

In the midst of all that vied for my attention, I rushed into a room to change an IV bag for a soft, pretzel-bent elderly woman with silky gray hair and papery skin. She had been incontinent, and I didn't have the time to bathe her and change the sheets. The sores on her body had no opportunity to heal because there weren't enough people on duty to give even the most basic of care. For some reason, it hit me hard that day. Maybe I was just the right kind of exhausted to make me as sensitive as an exposed nerve ending. I suddenly felt my efforts were the equivalent of pouring clear, fresh water onto a flat rock, watching it splatter and splash everywhere, with only a few tiny rivulets able to run off and penetrate where it was so badly needed. The supervisor couldn't provide any more help. I made it through that day, punched out, and never went back.

Still, I am proud of the work I did as a nurse. My sister-in-law has just begun nursing school. My two nieces will graduate from nursing school next year. I applaud them and others who may see it all very differently. I applaud their courage and tenacity. I applaud their hearts.

I'm 48 years old now, and I have not officially been a nurse for 18 years. By choice, I am no longer licensed and not practicing. Yet nursing is far more than a profession requiring licensure. The word *nurse* is an identity that is respected for its nobility of purpose. It is an identity that becomes you.

"Well, *you're* a nurse," friends will still sometimes say to me when they have a particular medical or health question, implying, "You should know." Never mind that I've been out of the business for years and that "If you don't use it, you lose it" applies to more than one area of living. There is a singularity of purpose associated with being a nurse. It's as if, when I became a nurse, no one could see any of the other facets of my personality. I was assumed into a role that defined me. It defines me still. "Once a nurse, always a nurse," they say.

For years I felt sad about leaving the nursing profession. I felt I'd failed in some fundamental way. As my spiritual quest deepened and I matured, over time I came to understand that there are many ways to be of service, that balance and boundaries are essential, and that we can only serve others well if our own basic needs are met. I came to understand that when we overempathize, we cannot be effective in changing a situation because we are then on an even keel with it. We must be above it to lift it up.

Home Visit

~

Elizabeth Tibbetts, RN

I didn't want to be
where a 90-year-old woman
rocked and looked out
on purple finches
at the feeder while bruises
slipped into sight from her sleeves:

the handling a gift from her son
who was gun-loving and volatile
as gasoline. Surely, he didn't learn
this from her, whose one remaining
joy was riding miles in the car,

the back of her boy's head before her,
and the fields and trees of her whole life
streaming by

her window. When did
his fury begin? When she bore him, one leg
too short, or 200 years before?

Now she cried every day and he said
it drove him crazy. The only quiet ones
were the skinny tom that urinated
from room to room and the son's wife,
who lay with her ruined back on the sofa

beneath the many eyes of Jesus Christ
looking out from all walls, clouds,
the Last Supper, and the cross.
I didn't want to tell them that no one
would come back to bathe

the old woman because of the gun,
and when I did, the son threw himself
to his feet, grabbed the rifle as if
by the hair, pointed it straight at me
a yard from my face, and screamed

as he snapped the chamber open
to show it was empty, that there
was not a godblasted thing to be afraid of.

Tough Jobs

~

Jo Ann Papich, AD

I READ WITH INTEREST a newspaper article about tough jobs. It stated that stressful jobs with low pay and lots of customer contact were the most likely to have high turnover rates. On the list of those who faced such stress were fast-food workers, meter readers, and nurses.

I am a nurse who quit. I started a new profession, and I am much happier—even though I make less money. Nursing is not a low-paying job, but it is stressful. You cannot have a bad day. You are responsible for the lives of other human beings. You are exposed to diseases. You are exposed to violent patients. You cannot give a Tylenol unless the doctor says so, but you can run a code. You also get blamed when a patient does not get what he or she wanted on a dinner tray. Administrators cut your staffing by one nurse per shift but expect the same quality of patient care from you—and they need you to work "extra."

If you are sick, if you or a loved one is in the hospital, please remember this. Nursing is one of the most difficult jobs there is. It challenges the nurse physically, mentally, emotionally, and spiritually. Remember that your nurse is overworked and tired. Remember that there is a shortage of people who are willing to put themselves through this much stress day after day. Please appreciate your nurse while you still have one.

Sondercommando

~

Anne Webster, RN

At a benefit for a wild bird sanctuary
people gnaw ribs to a blues band.
In chicken-wire cages pelicans squawk,
hop, peck at dry dirt. One teeters on
a single leg. One circles, dragging
its broken wing. Another, a chick in its beak,
beats the yellow body flat against a rock,
and it's 1961 again. I am 19,
a student nurse at Central State Hospital,
a jailer's keys hanging from my belt.
On the men's ward, psychopaths herd
schizophrenics through the showers,
shave the slack faces of catatonics.
In the day room a screened TV blares.
Patients stagger in orbit, rock in corners,

or argue with unheard voices while I play
gin rummy with joking psychos, soon
forgetting who has murdered, who has raped.
On Fridays patients from the chronic wards
pour into the gym. An inmate band saws
hillbilly tunes while I bump bellies
with Jesus, Napoleon, and sweaty men
who gallop or drool on my starched bib.
Other days I lead muttering women,
shuffling like Mother after her shock
treatments, to have their brains fried.
When the doctor turns on the juice,
I feel like a Jew herding loved ones
to the ovens at a death camp, holding down
a bucking arm or leg. At night, I wake
from a dream of maimed birds and wait
for a voice to order me to hand over
my keys, to join my kind in the pen.

From Nurse to Priest

~

Fr. Robert J. Kus, RN, PhD

THE PLACE WAS Cleveland, Ohio. The time was 1942. A young Bohemian American soldier named Bob and an Irish American RN called Pat decided to get married and have a baby. Unfortunately, the nurse had some condition that led her physicians to believe that if she were to become pregnant, she might become sick. In fact, they said, she might die. After carefully considering this information, Bob and Pat decided to take a chance on having a baby anyway.

As the pregnancy progressed, the physicians encouraged Pat to end her pregnancy because she was becoming ill. She would not hear of it. So, in the early-morning hours of March 30, 1943, Pat gave birth to a six-pound, four-ounce baby boy. That evening, she died. I was that baby, and I was named Robert James after my father and an uncle whose claim to fame was that he had laid the last brick in Cleveland's Terminal Tower.

Fast-forward 22 years. The place is a hallway outside the dining room at Cleveland Metropolitan General Hospital. A group of young graduates from the school of nursing are waiting to make their entry into the dining room that has been set up for a graduation ceremony. Among the 30-some graduates are three men, one of them me.

While I was waiting in line, two elderly people came up to me and asked if I was Robert Kus. When I said I was, they said, "Congratulations on your graduation! We have been following you for all these years." They gave me a small box with a bow on top and then disappeared. I never did learn who those people were.

When I opened the gift, I could hardly believe my eyes. There, in the box, was my mother's golden nursing pin from Cleveland's Saint Alexis Hospital School of Nursing. On the back was inscribed her maiden name. Thus began my journey into nursing.

From the earliest days in nursing school, I developed a very strong nursing identity. I was proud to be a nursing student, and I was passionate about the profession. I loved reading about heroic nurses, especially Catholic saints who were nurse-priests from days gone by, and about modern-day nurses who went to faraway lands and improved the quality of life of so many people.

So, at the age of 22, I began my career in a large county hospital as the weekend night-charge nurse of a gynecology unit while studying sociology full-time at a state university. At 23, I began teaching practical nursing to African American women in a Cleveland ghetto; and at 25, I began teaching in a state university while being a full-time student and part-time hospital RN. This pattern—full-time student, weekend night RN, and part-time university educator—was how I "grew up." Books, term papers, hospitals, and universities were my life.

For the next several years, I practiced every area of nursing except operating room and emergency room nursing, all the while teaching and studying. These years took me to Ohio, Montana, Washington State, Oklahoma, Iowa, Texas, Indiana, and North Carolina. Eventually I received a Ph.D. in sociology from the University of Montana and an M.S. in psychiatric/mental health nursing from the University of Oklahoma Health Sciences Center.

From 1982 to 1992, I taught at the University of Iowa College of Nursing, spent a summer teaching Ph.D. students at the University of Texas at Austin School of Nursing, and served as visiting scholar in Budapest, Hungary, and Prague, Czechoslovakia. In Prague, I had the honor of taking part in the Velvet Revolution, which brought down the Communist government in 1989.

Those years also took me to Europe and South America several times to do nursing research and present scholarly papers. I loved nursing. I loved teaching. I loved studying. But all the while, God was continually whispering to me, "I want you to become a priest." I first heard this whisper when I was about four years old, and I never doubted my destiny for a moment. Unfortunately, I had to wait for many years before God said, "Now's the time. Get ready for your seminary studies."

In 1998, at the age of 55, I was ordained a priest of the Diocese of Raleigh in North Carolina. I spent my first two years of priesthood in Wilmington, North Carolina, as a "parochial vicar," or associate pastor, of a large parish called Saint Mark. While there, I was affiliated with the School of Nursing and Department of Sociology at the University of North Carolina at Wilmington and taught a course called The Sociology of Birth and Death. Needless to say, my nursing background prepared me well for teaching this exciting and popular course.

From July 2000 to July 2006, I served as Pastor of Saint Catherine of Siena parish in Wake Forest, North Carolina, a rapidly growing suburb of Raleigh. (Wake Forest University, contrary to popular misconception, is not in Wake Forest, North Carolina. It was founded in Wake Forest but moved to Winston-Salem in 1956.) This rapidly growing parish of over 7,000 people had 42 percent of its population under the age of 18. It is sometimes called the "Cheerio Church," as people bring snacks to keep the kids quiet during mass.

From 2006 to the present, I have served as pastor of Saint Mary Catholic Church in Wilmington, a multi-cultural parish of around 6,000 people from every continent of the world except Antarctica. The parish has a strong social-justice base and serves over 10,000 poor persons a year with its social outreach ministry, AIDS ministry, and dental clinic. The exploding Hispanic community, filled with babies and children, is a constant joy to me. The youthful immigrants' enthusiasm and energy are contagious, and this bodes well for the future of the parish.

Sometimes, when people find out that I was primarily a psych nurse, they say, "Being a parish priest must be a whole lot different from being a psych nurse!" I joke that it is different in one great way. As a psych nurse, the people I served were called patients and were confined, and as a parish priest, the people I serve are called parishioners and are at large.

Actually, having a nursing background has enormous implications in my role as priest. Priests enter into people's lives in most intimate ways and at most critical life events—births, deaths, weddings, divorces, and milestone celebrations such as baptisms and First Communions. The good old communication skills that I learned as a nursing student serve to help my parishioners open up in amazing ways. Empathy, additive empathy, self-disclosure, confrontation, purposeful questioning, and so on are all like sparkling jewels for both priest and nurse. Although people trust nurses readily, I find they trust priests even more. People know, for example, that priests would give their lives rather than divulge information they receive in the Sacrament of Reconciliation.

The greatest communication skill I have at my disposal as a nurse-priest, though, is the skill of listening, really listening. This includes not just hearing what people are saying but also identifying how they are saying it. What is their body language? What is the real issue? I know that, quite often, what people begin to talk about is not what really is on their mind. Rather, they have to talk about "safe" things first before getting down to the heart of the problem. When I visit the Lower Cape Fear Hospice Center, for example, people often begin by telling me about their parish and their families. As I listen, though, they begin to express their fears of the afterlife and guilt from past transgressions.

Once these fears are out in the open, I am able to provide some reassurance of God's infinite mercy and love.

As a parish priest, I counsel people with a gamut of life problems: spouse abuse, alcoholism and other forms of drug addiction, financial problems, infidelity, constant anger, loss of a job, death of a loved one, loss of family, mental and physical illness, spiritual maladies such as scrupulosity, vocational uncertainties, and the like. Because of my background in nursing, especially psychiatric/mental health and chemical dependency nursing, I am able to counsel wisely and make intelligent referrals to family counselors, personal counselors, financial help agencies, attorneys, physicians, social workers, and the like.

Being an RN also gains me instant entrée into the world of nursing. For example, when I make hospital visits to ICUs or other areas that have strictly limited access to outsiders, I mention to the RNs that I'm an RN too; at that point they not only invite me in but also share things about the patients that they would never share with other kinds of visitors. When I was visiting a hospital in Uganda, East Africa, for example, the director of nursing was initially very polite and formal toward me as a priest. When she learned that I was truly an RN even though I'm a man—a strange concept in Uganda—she personally took me under her wing and gave me the grand tour.

Instant camaraderie between nurses is something that can also be found outside hospital settings. Once, for example, I was in West Berlin to present a couple of addiction papers just before the two Germanys were to be reunited. I was walking toward a bus stop that I hoped would take me to the Reichstag, where the conference was. I went up to someone and asked if this was the correct way to get to where I was going, hoping that he could speak English. An African American woman came dashing toward me and said, "You're an American! Thank God! I'm lost, and this is the first time I've ever been lost in a foreign language!" I learned she was an RN also, and that she was presenting a paper at the same conference I was. The rest of the week we became best buddies.

Another great thing that I have taken from nursing and applied to pastoral care is the nursing process: assessment, diagnosis, outcome identification, planning, implementation, and evaluation. This model serves me well in virtually any situation in dealing with staff or parishioner problems.

Being an RN also helps in crisis situations, situations where others may fall apart. In fact, I have found in my life, and in the lives of many other RNs, that we often function *better* in crisis situations than in ordinary situations. At Saint Catherine's, for example, the director of religious education (DRE) was also an RN. Whenever there was a crisis—something that can occur at the drop of a hat in a 7,000-member parish—the DRE was able to spring into action. I had total trust that she could and would handle the situation, get help if she needed it, and report back to me on the solution. Many times I would have to call on this DRE when I was tied up with other duties to handle an agitated, disturbed, or angry person who came into the office.

Having practiced nursing all over the United States and visited many foreign countries has prepared me well for dealing with people from different cultures. Cultural diversity is something I treasure. That is a good thing, for people in my parish come from more than 50 nations of the world. I especially treasure the Hispanic community of my parish, a community that composes about one-third of the congregation. Because most of our Hispanic community is Mexican, there are a wide variety of celebrations at Saint Catherine's such as *quinceañeras* (for 15-year-old girls), *presentaciónes en el templo* (for 3-year-old children), and ceremonies of the *lazo* (lasso) and *arras* (coins) at weddings. There are also processions of many types, especially for Our Lady of Guadalupe, and we decorate an *altar de muertos* (altar of the dead) for November 1 and 2.

Finally, I learned early on in my nursing career that even the most difficult and challenging patient is easy compared to a staff member who becomes problematic. This is definitely true in the parish setting; the grief caused by problematic parishioners cannot begin to compare to that caused by staff members who have gone sour. I imagine that is true in any type of social organization. One staff member in a former parish, for example, had a highly negative presentation of self and outlook on life. No matter how cheerful the staff was, the spirits of the group dropped the moment this person entered the room. The person was like a sponge that drained joy and cheer and life from whatever group she found herself in. Fortunately, the woman resigned and was replaced by a joyful type of person whom all the staff treasured.

As I look back on my life, I see how God was leading me at every step of the way. I did not understand why, since I wanted to be a priest from the time I was four, God made me wait so long. But now I see that God had a plan, and that everything I have experienced was to prepare me for a special priesthood. I now see, for example, how taking college courses in acting was so helpful in allowing me to avoid stage fright as a parish priest who speaks before 2,000 people every weekend. I now see how all the courses in writing were actually preparing me to write a homily every week, plus my columns for two Spanish-speaking magazines and daily radio reflection program. But I especially treasure all I learned in nursing, for from nursing I became the kind of priest I am today. What nursing has given me is limitless.

Would I encourage others to enter nursing? Of course! As a matter of fact, I actively and frequently recruit men and women into nursing in my parish work. To be a nurse is one of the noblest callings a person can have. I thank God every day for the privilege of being part of the company of nurses.

CEUs Before
the Hurricane

~

Sally Bellerose, RN

A couple of 64-hour weeks
in yet another nursing-shortage summer
buys me a ticket to a convention in New Orleans.
Six RNs and an EMT
think we've seen it all until we
stop at a bar on Bourbon Street.

Inside, a woman lies naked on a mirror.
Her image hangs over herself
on another mirror suspended
at a well-calculated angle.
She's not a subject on a slide;
still we peer like first-year students,

eyes wide, hands behind our backs,
straining to make sense of what we see.

I can't see the sex in it.
Could be her, could be me.
Who is too professional?
What I see is a woman bored
with labor, like I am, weary
of my job's demands.

She sweats like an aerobics instructor.
Her moves have too much pattern
to be the real thing. Too little
old-fashioned, excited Brownian
motion, vaguely recalled,
through the lens of nursing school.

Still, the place is packed.
She's getting the job done.
Her eyes roam from patron to patron.
Eventually her gaze lands on me.

Her eyes are laughing.
Do they see I admire hard work?
She smiles, winks, and I feel chosen.
I want to tell her I'm a nurse,
I work hard too. I want to ask her how
to bounce back,
keep my eyes alive,
make them speak
to the people my body is moving for?

But her eyes go
to another patient—I mean patron—
ten dollars' worth, the cover charge,
then move on.

How I Found
My Way Back

❦

Patty Smith Hall, RN

O N   T H A T   N O V E M B E R morning I stared at the legal-sized envelope clutched in my hands, knowing that the contents would finally free me from the shackles of bitterness I'd been wearing these last few years.

The renewal form for my nursing license.

I traced the return address on the envelope. Ten years ago, I would never have considered the possibility of giving up my license. As anyone who has ever sat for the state boards would know, relinquishing the legal ability to practice nursing borders on insanity. But that morning, I saw it as the final step toward my healing, a painful process that had started years earlier when I was attacked by a patient.

He didn't mean to hurt me, the post-op patient in bed 419. Although ours was not a surgical floor, he was assigned to a room at the end of our hall as a favor to one of the doctors on staff. No one expected him to have a drug-induced psychotic episode, least of all a novice nurse like me. And I would never have thought that night would be my last on the floor as a nurse.

But not as a patient.

Unbelievable pain seared a trail across my buttocks and down my right leg, ending behind my knee. My toes and the bottom of my foot suddenly went numb and cold. Later we would learn that the force of the attack had dislocated my hip bones and ruptured a series of discs in my lower back. The doctors reacted conservatively, treating me with rest, drugs, and traction, but soon it became clear that surgery was my only option.

No one ever sat me down and told me about the possible long-term effects of my injuries, and to be honest, I never considered it. I thought I would have the affected discs repaired, recuperate for a couple of months, and then get on with my life. It wasn't until the day after my surgery, while I drifted in and out of sleep, that I learned the full extent of my injuries.

Profound nerve damage. Chronic pain with periods of paralysis.

"She'll never be able to work as a nurse again."

Even in my semiconscious state, I felt my heart shuttering. Not be a nurse? I couldn't fathom the idea. Why would God allow this to happen to me, especially after all the study and hardship I went through to get my degree? I wanted to scream but couldn't find my voice.

I continued to heal. And as my body began to return to normal, so did my will. I decided not to take the doctor's prognosis lying down. I would fight for my career.

The first few weeks post-op were filled with periods of physical therapy, insurance negotiations, and depression. I couldn't eat and lost so much weight that the visiting nurse thought I had an eating disorder. The hospital and my doctors couldn't agree on what kind of work I could do, so I soon found myself without a job.

I started searching the want ads, but each interview ended in disappointment. No one would hire an inexperienced nurse with my medical history. Some of my friends suggested that I keep my back problems a secret, but I couldn't do that and live with myself.

At 23, I was unemployable.

Six months and hundreds of résumés later, I was offered a position at a research facility. For the next seven years I worked in pediatric research, teaching parents care for their high-risk infants. I was finally doing the kind of work God had called me to do.

But physically, I wasn't doing so well. I tried to pretend everything was okay, laughing over the times I'd trip over my numb foot and ignoring the pain running across my hip and down my leg. It was only when I began to fall consistently that I contacted a doctor.

An alphabet of tests followed—MRIs, CAT scans, EMGs. Days later, the doctor had a verdict: stenosis of the spinal column, extensive nerve damage, more ruptured discs. My nursing career was officially over.

But my heart wouldn't let go. Nursing was who I was. God wouldn't do this to me, would he? Not when I had followed his calling. If my career was gone, what did that mean for me? I was ashamed of my disability, believing it made me less of a person.

In my anger, I backed away from family and friends. Why would they want to have anything to do with a 29-year-old cripple? Our home became a battlefield as I slipped further into depression. My husband and I fought constantly. One evening he came home to his packed clothes and my demand that he leave.

My world imploded.

"Please get help," my parents said.

I agreed to meet with a counselor. She was nice enough, asking questions and listening to me as I rambled on nervously. Those sessions helped me understand the anger that had been brewing inside me since the accident. And I finally learned the answer to my question of why this had happened to me.

Why not?

I had a choice. I could live my life sitting at home, dealing with the pain that stayed with me every moment of every day. Or I could get involved in the world around me. Would the pain go away? No, but the empty feeling of not taking charge of my life would.

Within a year, I was involved in my community—substitute teaching, volunteer work. Although I still lived in pain, I had found a life worth living.

So on that morning in November when I held that envelope in my hands, I had a choice: hang on to the past, or embrace the new future God had in store for me. I tossed the envelope into the garbage can.

My healing was complete. I was finally free.

My Nontraditional Choice

~

Holly Anderson, RN, CCM

Five years ago I began my journey into the world of nursing. But let me start from the beginning. . . .

I decided to do this whole career thing in reverse—I opted to have children first, raise them, and then return to school. At age 41, I began the journey that would lead me to the career choice I had made from early childhood: I wanted to be a nurse.

Genetics probably played a part in my decision, since both my grandmother and my uncle were nurses. All I know is that I was determined to get my degree and it couldn't happen quickly enough. I signed up for the required classes and entered the nursing program a year earlier than I'd anticipated, overjoyed, eager and ready to jump in.

In May 2000, I was granted the degree I dreamed of for so long. Happy to have successfully made it this far, I began the search for the "perfect job" in nursing. The trouble with that idealistic plan was—and I was clueless here—that there is no such animal. Instructors had advised the best place to launch from would be a medical-surgical unit in a hospital setting in order to obtain a well-rounded experience. I applied at a facility about half an hour's drive from home and was offered a position as a graduate nurse on a medical-surgical/pediatric unit. I was ecstatic, ready to springboard into the realm of saving the world from the evils of disease processes.

Much to my disappointment, things were not at all as I had anticipated they would be. Lo and behold, unbeknownst to me, I had just entered a dog-eat-dog world, one that would forever change my point of view concerning this profession. I soon discovered that the clinical aspect of school was no preparation for the real world of hospital nursing, which included 14-hour nights (12 hours on the floor, 2 hours of catch-up charting), increasing patient loads, mandatory call shifts, hospital politics, and the more seasoned nurses consuming their progeny.

Not wanting to become a nursing casualty by continuing to work on a unit I felt was not a good fit for me, I turned to a field in which I thought I would excel: obstetrical nursing. After all, I was a mother! I had lived through four deliveries myself, and now with my nursing degree to support me, surely I could withstand the onslaughts of whatever might come my way. Wrong again.

So my quest continued. Nine months here, a year and a half there, I was always seeking and searching, never finding my niche in this profession. Five years later, just as I was ready to throw in the towel and leave the field of nursing altogether, my search led me to an area of nursing I had no idea existed: theme park nursing. What a novel idea! Who ever heard of such a thing? My mind was racing. My youngest daughter had just graduated from vocational school and accepted a position in another state, so I was ready to give nursing one last try. The theme park was located in another state, 1,100 miles from home. Always having had an insatiable desire for adventure, I convinced my dear sweet husband of 31 years that this was only for the summer and that I would return home by fall. I assured him he could visit whenever he wanted to, and I would come home as time allowed. I truly felt this was the answer for me, and I just had to give it a shot (pardon the pun). Long story short, I applied, interviewed, was hired, and headed for Los Angeles.

Never in my life would I have dreamed that my initial orientation would consist of riding rides and viewing attractions. What fun my former colleagues were missing out on! This was incredible! I soon learned how to navigate the park, learned which rides were the most apt to hazard, and what a foreign tourist was asking for if he requested paracetamol (a.k.a. acetaminophen, or Tylenol). This was too good to be true!

My summer ended all too quickly, and before I knew it, it was time to return home. Knowing my choices were few, I once again returned to bedside nursing, dreading each and every moment of what I knew lay ahead. I came back to earth with a thud.

Trying my best to complete each day with a smile, I decided I could no longer bear the thought of 12-hour shifts, increasing patient-to-nurse ratios, and long nights. My stomach hurt every time I drove into the parking lot at work. I had gotten a taste of my perfect job in nursing and was miserable that I had only been able to have the experience for a mere summer. I devoted a portion of each day to searching the Internet, hoping against hope to find something comparable to what I had experienced, but alas, it was not to be found. There just were no major theme parks that needed RNs in Colorado. After six months I turned once again to jobs in the Los Angeles area, applied to work for a major studio, and arranged to fly out for an interview. Additionally a former coworker had given me a lead on a job in another facet of nursing I had not yet discovered: case management. Suffice it to say that I was scheduled for two interviews in Los Angeles and was offered a position with an insurance company as a complex case manager. Although the setting was different from what I had experienced during the previous summer months, I was (and still am) intrigued by it. Interestingly, the studio to which I had applied offered me a per diem position as well; I accepted both jobs and, as a result, have decided to remain in the nursing profession.

In conclusion, the past year has shown me that rather than walking away from a profession that has been severely impacted by personnel shortages, there are still areas of the field to explore. My purpose in submitting this essay is to offer encouragement to my fellow nurses who are feeling burned out, unfulfilled, or disappointed. I want to share the good news that there are options available. It may require something of you (my husband and I sold our home in beautiful Colorado and relocated to Southern California), but if you are patient and persistent, you never know when that window of opportunity in nursing will open for you!

I Could Have Been a Rock Star

~

Jim Cardwell, RN

I could have been a rock star
    then died of an overdose,
    gone down in a plane,
    or been stalked by homicidal fans.
A buckaroo
    bucked off, bruised, ofttimes broken,
    only able to count to ten
    by using both hands and one foot.
An Iowa farmer
    poisoned by pesticides
    or chewed up in my own feed grinder
    if not foreclosed on first.
Perhaps a poet
    then died a drunk at 39,

been stabbed by a jealous lover,
or committed suicide over rejection.

I should quit now.
I'm disgusted
by habitually
hostile, noncompliant patients
irresponsibly expecting
that some magic telemarket medicine
will cure lifelong self-abuse
then exploding at me when told
"That myth died with Disney."
And like Walt,
those pagans await that cryonic age
when ruined bodies can be
revived,
repaired, and ruined again.

But where will I find a vocation
to match my difficult demeanor,
allowing my attitudes and abilities
free rein of expression?
Where my best work is appreciated,
without fear of repercussion,
not expected every time?
Where being 99.9 percent right
can't cost me a career?
Where death
Is not the outcome of a really bad day?

The Lungs Are the Organ of Sorrow

~

Michelle Ashley

YOU'VE ALWAYS BEEN there for me. Steady and reliable. Breathe in. Breathe out. Like skin, you are exposed to the environment in an intimate way. Breathe in. Breathe out. I go to a wild party, you go to a wild party. Breathe in. Breathe out. I go to a haunted house with a smoke machine—you go there too. Breathe in. Breathe out. I spend a day at the beach and you take in the salty air too. Breathe in. Breathe out. I go running next to the buses spewing diesel fumes and you are dragged along too. Breathe in. Breathe out. Like clockwork. I never have to think twice. I never doubt your existence; I could not imagine your not being there. Breathe in. Breathe out. And in my presumption I forget your importance.

"YOU HAVE A tumor in your middle right lobe, and you need further diagnostic tests," I was told. How could you have left me? How could you have betrayed me? Breathe in. Breathe out. Even though I was shocked and angry with you, you stuck with me while I waited those three months for the test. Breathe in. Breathe out. And I realized how important you were to me. Breathe in. Breathe out. And I had neglected not only you but other parts of my body as well. Breathe in. Breathe out. And neglected even my own feelings and fears. Breathe in. Breathe out.

"IT HASN'T GROWN any more, and it is a benign tumor." Breathe in. Breathe out. Now the take-home message is to pay more attention to what you try to tell me. Breathe in. Breathe out. We all have a story to tell, and your story is a reflection of your relationship with me. Breathe in. Breathe out. I will spend more time focusing on you and let the thoughts become more constructive with each breath. Breathe in. Breathe out. And, with any luck, we will spend our days with each other and fill them with memories as we grow old together. Breathe in. Breathe out. And what did that nurse tell the crowd at a rally years ago? Breathe in. Breathe out. "We nurses are there when you take your first breath"—breathe in—"and we are there when you take your last"—breathe out.

Chest Clippers

~

Kathryn Gahl, BSN, BS, RN

THE DEAD OF night. 1975. The surgical intensive care unit at Johns Hopkins Hospital. A tech sitting at the monitors sees V-tach in room 4. He pushes a red button and cries, "Code Blue!" Suddenly, room 4 crowds with two residents, two interns, two RNs, one GN, and a different tech. Pumping and thumping begins on the patient, a man with a thick shock of white hair and a year-round tan. Drugs are mainlined. A long needle shoots intracardiac epinephrine straight into the right ventricle. The clock ticks, and I, the recorder, know how many interminable minutes we have been at this—with no response. Another machine rumbles into the room; it contains the life-giving paddles. "Stand back!" a resident yells. The army of caregivers clears the bed. Our man is shocked, but his heart won't respond.

More drugs and more CPR until the senior resident screams, "Chest clippers!" The clippers appear like shears for a wise gardener. But the senior resident hands them to the junior resident. "Go ahead," the senior one says. "It's the last hope." The junior resident snips through the staples. The staples pop one at a time until we peer into the man's airless chest cavity. Immediately, the junior resident begins open-heart massage. *Squeeze, squeeze, come on, damn it, please.* The patient is up to his neck in blood, his 62-year-old heart like a shabby sponge, soft and yielding. The resident stops the massage. He looks at the monitor. Nothing. He resumes with all the grit of a cook tenderizing roundsteak. After 20 minutes, he asks me if I want to do it. Woozy and sleep-deprived, I glove up and soon cradle the man's heart in my hands.

I squeeze. The heart, larger than my shaky hand, leaks more blood. It is like clay—stiff and with much more mass than I expect. I remember the first time I milked a cow after watching my father's strong hands squeeze, squeeze, first one teat, then the other, as pale blue milk hit the pail in 2/4 time. I tried then. I try now. Both processes require more strength than I have. Defeated, I thank the resident, and withdraw my bloody gloved hands. He resumes.

I am a new nurse, this my first job—hence the night shift. Another intern and I watch in awe, gullible, believing that the man will be saved. The intern, an undergrad philosophy major, asks if I know about the theory of the last heartbeat. I do not. He explains that each of us are born with a certain number of heartbeats. "If you use up yours in jogging or in playing tennis, well, then you go earlier." He says he will use his judiciously, none of that heavy-duty exercise. We look at the suntanned man while the resident squeezes the hell out of his heart. The intern shrugs, certain there are no beats left in the patient's sinus node. Then silence enters the room. It is the recognition that sometime during the two-and-a-half-hour show, the heart-attack man in the bed in room 4 left us like a shooting star.

At change of shift in the morning, a day RN learns of the night's excitement.

"Bastards," she says. "They were just having fun."

One of the residents hears her remark. "Curing is part of the care," he says.

"Caring is part of the cure," I reply, thinking of the family's collective heartache. But the voice inside me is downtrodden and dumb. And I have the first of many repetitive thoughts: How can I stay in nursing? How can I reconcile the difference between doctoring and nursing?

AFTER ONE YEAR, I left the high-wire tension of Johns Hopkins SICU. I searched to find a place with fewer heroics and less technology. That summer, I worked as a Girl Scout camp nurse, dealing with two seventh-graders who swallowed poison because they did not want to walk the Appalachian Trail. In autumn, I worked in a scaled-down ICU at Church Hospital, a place for the indigent next to Hopkins. Then I moved back to Wisconsin to work in emergency and medical-surgical units. I substitute-taught at the local technical college. I wrote feature articles for local newspapers, using the English degree I'd earned before I went into nursing. And then, after the birth of my children, I found my niche in obstetrics. I stayed in that arena for two decades because there, for me, doctoring and nursing melded. There we worked together to see a star born. Looking back, I see how much I loved beginnings and how lousy I was with endings.

That's probably why now, as a full-time writer, I never know how the short story, poem, novel, or children's book I write is going to end. There is risk and excitement in the unknown, the fact that life is rich and unpredictable, no matter what reason we climb out of bed every day and begin anew.

One on One with Dylan Thomas

~

Theodore Deppe, RN, MFA

I'm taking my break outside the detox unit,
      watching a junkie shoot baskets in the parking lot,
admiring the lazy arc and swish of her 15-footers,

     when a scrap of last night's dream returns:

I'm one on one with Dylan Thomas,
        who drops his shoulder
    and drives baseline, reversing his layup so the ball
spins on the rim and drops in.

He's short and slow and
   impossible to guard:
      feint to the right, three quick steps to the basket
         before he shovel-flips
  the ball around me.

Maybe it's time to find another job.
Maybe the last time I made a difference here
    is months past, before this place began to
        traffic in quick cures.

Years ago, Coach Froligher ordered me to quit
    our high school production of Dylan's *Under Milk Wood.*
        Coach,
    quietly intense, got what he wanted
                by speaking so softly his players leaned

toward him, off balance, to hear.
    He wanted me to think
        only of the next game,
            wanted everything to ride on it.

Sometimes I tell the story of why I quit the team
    as though it began
            my present life,
Dylan's voice echoing in mine as I strode off court,
    though I imagine
        my last words to Coach were
                high-pitched
        and graceless, abject stubbornness pressed to decide.

This junkie—a woman named Noni I've only talked with once,
    whose habits and boyfriend force her to turn tricks—
                has asked an orderly for a light.
I like the way the ball's release and cigarette's removal from her
    lips
        are one motion, her deft handling of
                awkward transitions, how she exhales and

rebounds an errant shot, fires again,
>> two-hand jumper, this one
> kissing
>> the rim, swirling through before the long drag's
>> prompt reward.

What could I say
> that would help her walk out
>> next time she's ordered to sell herself
> for a nickel bag?

"Begin at the beginning," Dylan intones,
> the Caedmon recording I bought
bringing back the play's smoke-lit opening night,
>> a few months before his death.

Words can't save us
> though I walked off court, however tongue-tied,
>> intoxicated
>> by the slap and surge of slow vowels.
This must be the boyfriend,
>> long-sleeved on a sweltering day,
> come to take Noni on pass.

>> Let him tell Noni
one too many times,
> "You'll never be anything
> but a strung-out whore."

Let him break
> her nose again, if that's what it takes.

Too long I've fought against
    becoming one thing or the other:

            all right, damn it, force us to choose.

Documenting the
Shades of Gray

~

Jenna Rindo, RN

I STOOD, HESITATING AND nervous, outside the closed door of my first official patient's room at the Medical College of Virginia Hospital in Richmond. I was faced with my first solo decision as a student nurse. Did I knock or just barge right in to collect the patient's vitals and begin my head-to-toe assessment early that Monday morning?

Perhaps I should have taken that moment as an ominous sign. Nursing proved not to be a career for which I was well suited in the long haul. Twenty years later, and I can't recall that first patient's name or diagnosis—though at the time I'm certain I had developed an extensive care plan for him—with each of his medications on a drug card, fluorescent highlights noting side effects, expected dosage, and method of action. I was starting my first clinical rotation on a medical-surgical floor and was just beginning to question my decision to get my bachelor of science in nursing.

Leaving the safety of the classroom, with its predictable paper-and-pencil exams and assignments, for the hands-on procedures and assessments involved in the clinical rotations took me way out of my comfort zone. My grandpa would have simply stated I was book smart but not horse smart. (He worked in the powder plant outside Blacksburg, Virginia, but made extra money buying, selling, and trading horses.) I handled the intellectual challenges of the math and science courses and the nursing board exam with no problem. But when it came time to apply my knowledge on ill and suffering humans, I always doubted myself to one extent or another.

I graduated in 1987 and had thousands of dollars of student loans to pay back. I didn't really dare to admit to anyone (even myself) that my career choice might be completely wrong. To do so seemed unthinkable, along the same lines as standing someone up at the wedding altar. I had no trouble getting a job in the area of my choice, which was pediatric special care, and I bravely reported for duty—wearing a uniform or street clothes with a full-length lab coat as my contract specified.

I worked as a registered nurse in pediatric units at hospitals in Virginia, Florida, and Wisconsin for seven years. Though I loved certain aspects of hospital nursing, if I'm honest I'll admit that I never achieved the level of confidence it takes to feel that elusive sense known as job satisfaction. Certainly I mastered the more concrete nursing procedures and eventually could perform them automatically. I saw that flash of yellow or amber-colored urine in the plastic tubing of a Foley catheter and knew I was "in." I counted apical pulse rates and recorded digital temperatures. I weighed diapers dry and wet to ascertain intake and output. Yet hundreds of other assessment areas were much less concrete and more subject to interpretation. I would listen to lung sounds again and again—did I hear subtle crackles in the lower left lobe? How could those lips look slightly cyanotic when the pulse oximeter clearly read 97 percent? Seasoned nurses have a sixth sense that tells them when something doesn't look or feel right about a patient. I perceived them as having some sort of special power to foresee and then ward off a patient crash or crisis—a power that I felt I clearly lacked.

I never seemed able to breeze in, assess and document my findings, administer meds, perform wound care or trach care, and change sterile central line tubing with the necessary confidence required. I questioned my five senses and my ability to perform procedures quickly enough. I worried way too much about everything and anything. I called to check on certain patients long after my shift ended and I should have been sleeping soundly. I lived in fear of being the only nurse present when a critical patient was admitted. Each time the charge nurse left for a cigarette break, I was convinced that one of her patients would crash and I would be left alone to deal with it.

I'll never forget the first time one of my patients died. The code was carried out according to procedure, his condition had been deteriorating for days, and yet somehow I still felt completely defeated. The death of this patient,

I thought, was some sort of blatant failure on my part. Calling the parents and readying the body of this six-month-old boy—who had lived all his life in the hospital on a ventilator, never unconnected from a maze of internal lines and monitors—were two of the most difficult things I've ever done. By the time the mother came in, my shift had ended and the day shift had taken over. I lurked at the nurses' station instead of clocking out or doing what I should have done, which was to rush over to the mother and cry right along with her. I realize my cowardly mistake years later now that I am a mother.

I could go on and on trying to explain my nursing strengths and weaknesses. I could quote all the wonderful comments documented by parents on their exit surveys. I developed a level of comfort with long-term patients and their family members. I fell in love with the babies and toddlers who had no family. I contemplated adopting certain patients or at the very least becoming their foster parent. I struggled to maintain the balance between maternal instinct and professional distance. Later, when I had my first child, I seemed to struggle with leaving my clinical skills at the hospital and letting my maternal gut take control. I found myself counting my daughter's respiratory rate as she slept. I felt almost guilty as I tossed her heavy wet diapers into the trash without weighing them on a gram scale. My role as a mom and a registered nurse never developed clear boundaries. I had too much empathy at work, and I worried way too much at home about each childhood illness and slight drop off the growth-chart curve. Why wasn't she in the 50th percentile or above for height and weight? Was my breast milk lacking at some cellular level? It killed me not to be able to measure in ounces her intake at each feeding.

My decision to leave nursing was complicated and yet also a huge relief. If I had to explain it to someone in a sentence or less, I would simply say I always had a slightly sick feeling in my gut an hour or two before it was time to go to work. It didn't seem to matter if I was on a run of graveyard shifts or rotating between first and second shifts. I always felt a mild unrest—a sense of foreboding knowing I had to work. There was always the knowledge that anything could happen during a shift—be it 8 or 12 hours. A patient's condition could rapidly deteriorate; new admits could come through the door at any time; or someone on the next shift could call in sick, and if central administration couldn't find a replacement I'd stay to pull a double. I never fully adjusted to the uncertainties involved in critical hospital nursing. I finally allowed myself to listen to my gut feelings and admit I had made a mistake. Maybe I was influenced by the nursing shortage of the 1980s or trying to prove something to my own parents, who had confessed misgivings about my plan to go into nursing from the onset.

After working as a nurse full-time for five years, I decided to cut back to part-time work on a pediatric floor at the local hospital so that I could go back to school to obtain my elementary teaching certification. Though the 18 weeks of student teaching were challenging and I experienced moments of frustration and self-doubt, I never once reached the point of feeling physically sick. I currently teach English as a second language to Hmong, Arabic, and Spanish students. Teaching requires a level of self-reflection and planning that hospital nursing did not accommodate. As a teacher, I've gained control of my daily schedule, the resources and methods I use to teach different students different subjects, and the amount and kinds of assessment records I maintain. I create the physical classroom space and the safe atmosphere necessary for the risks involved in learning a new language. I've been teaching in this setting for 11 years and feel a level of comfort I never reached in nursing. Pediatric nursing and teaching overlap in many ways. Both require flexibility, patience, and ongoing assessment of the subtle clues and nuances children send. Teaching affords me the luxury of long-term relationships and the opportunity to see my students' physical, emotional, and intellectual growth. When I was a pediatric nurse, my patients were discharged once they reached a stable level of wellness.

I have great admiration and appreciation for nurses, as well as respect for all people willing to make changes in their vocations and start over as nontraditional students in any field. I could end with any number of clichés along the lines of "Experience is the best teacher" or "Always listen to your gut feelings." It seems that some people tend to see the world in clearly contrasted black-and-white, while others (myself included) always find infinite shades of gray. The things that matter most—the larger questions around faith, relationships, and vocation—require each of us to find our own way of seeing clearly.

Home Visits

~

Paula Sergi, BSN, MFA

No wonder I paused at their doorsteps,
measuring the distance between us:
my shining young skin, my white teeth, white shoes,
my crisp jacket, new job, fresh breath.
Before the knock I'd hesitate, checking their charts
for the wound where the pressure of time
had worn holes in their skins.

Most were near the end of their unpeeling,
shedding layers of memory and money.
On the other side of their doors, the acrid
ammonia of urine melted in their bedding,
their trousers and stockings. Drainage-soaked
gauzes trailed behind as they shuffled
to answer the bell.

I wrote care plans directing my visits,
mapping the way those wounds would heal,
from the outside in, and listed what I'd use
to fill them: ointments and creams,
plastic sheets like skin itself glued over
their oozing gaps. Orange-colored scrubs
or vinegar. Even sugar sprinkled on like faith.

With my little healer's tools I listened to the pressure
of blood against their vessels as their corpuscles tried
to escape. Catheters drained their amber urine
and plugged up and had to be plumbed. Urine bags
hung like handbags over walkers or bed rails.
I poured their pills into plastic cups, marking
time on calendars big as their kitchen tables.

But I was distracted: the corners of their homes,
the cobwebs and cuckoo clocks, veneered end tables,
scratched woodwork, what the windowsill
figurines could say. Sometimes I'd hear about
lovely mothers, the children they never saw again.
And when the hour was up, I'd shout
my instructions and leave.

It's not that I didn't want to touch them.
We had no idea, back then, about age
passing itself on. It's taken years
for me to recognize a skin that won't
bounce back, a stuttered gait on icy walks,
elusive words that hide behind
the floaters in my eyes. Once in a while

I'd see it when I washed their bony backs,
a used-up body about to lift off
with scapular wings. The glitter of dust motes
above their birdlike heads as they sat
by their windows watching me coming
and going, still lives of another kind. Above
little cloud-tufts of hair, halos for the almost dead.

Boy with Many Hats

~

Elizabeth Jane Hill, RN

SAM LOVED TO try on all sorts of hats. He'd put on a new one, come up close to someone's face, and stare straight in that person's eyes until he or she acknowledged how handsome he looked. Though he had no voice because of his tracheostomy tube, he'd make squeaks and squawks of delight to get a person's attention.

I love those last two pictures taken of him. In one, he's wearing his Santa Claus stocking hat. In the other, he dons his mom's big black cowboy hat. In Santa's hat, he had both arms raised with hands and fingers fully extended, his signature open-mouthed smile aglow as if shouting "Hooray!" Then wearing Mom's oversized cowboy ten-gallon, he became a handsome dude, his broad, full-lipped grin and sparkling blue eyes accentuating the look.

His passing happened so suddenly and absolutely there was nothing anyone could do to bring him back that fifth day after Christmas. His leaving left a gaping hole in the heart of the family structure as well as the healthcare team centered around the triplets.

It was so unexpected, as Sam was the most outwardly robust of the three boys, essentially age-appropriate physically and cognitively. He'd been doing so well. He was, along with another of his brothers, in the beginning stages of the decannulation process (removal of the tracheotomy tube). It was two and a half years since their birth at 25 weeks gestation, a minute-by-minute existence of intensive therapies and 24-hour home nursing care.

LIKE MANY OTHER premature infants, all three had required tracheotomies and mechanical ventilation within a few months of life because their immature lungs had developed a life-threatening condition called bronchopulmonary dysplasia.

Sam and one of his brothers had finally progressed enough to be off their ventilators, and they were catching up physically with the help of various therapies. The third and smallest brother would still need months more of full-time mechanical ventilation and intensive therapies to progress as far. However, it was nothing short of a miracle that this small one, like his brothers, was able to be cared for at home, where he was making good strides.

With 24-hour private-duty nursing care and with various therapies required every day for each boy, the house was a bustling place with all manner of beeps and alarms sounding every few minutes. Although their cribs were situated in the living room, the boys and their equipment took over every room in the house.

For many of us, there was little chance for closure after Sam's passing. The family, understandably, needed privacy in their decisions and grieving process. However, with two surviving but medically fragile boys remaining at home to care for, along with all the support people, nurses, equipment, and therapies required daily, privacy and time were scarce indeed.

In my early days as a pediatric nurse, I had worked with many terminally ill children. In particular, it was those with cystic fibrosis who had profoundly affected me, and ultimately had led me into making sculpture as a means to cope with my grief and burnout when they passed. I had witnessed in many of these children a depth of wisdom and fullness of spirituality usually associated with the elderly. Most would orchestrate their leaving, careful to prepare their families for the loss and to reassure them in the process. Youngsters as young as seven or eight would hold on until their loved ones were able to release them.

Over the years, these experiences informed and inspired my sculpture-making, helping to open and develop my own spirituality. Making sculptures and teaching others to sculpt not only became my spiritual practice but ultimately led me to return to nursing after nearly 20 years of absence from the field. In the process, my sculpture career evolved into community-based arts, based in education and healing through creativity.

I had not carved stone in nearly ten years when I began *Boy with Many Hats.* My more recent works had been of softer materials and subject matter, mostly puppets and dolls that I perform with. However, as this work was to be a memorial in Sam's honor, limestone it had to be. Limestone is a common stone with a lovely texture that holds paints very well while visually retaining its stone qualities. Unlike the tighter and harder surface of marble, limestone is not so easily transformed into a fleshy look.

In my way of thinking about this memorial, the image needed to be that of a "stone boy," as opposed to a stone transformed into a boy of flesh. Sam's life on earth was now "carved in stone," and only chiseling and grinding stone could suffice to describe the pain of his loss.

It was summer. I set up a tent in my backyard, and began. Next to me was a board full of copied pictures of Sam from which to work. I conceived the carving as a totem, made up of three block-cut stacked stones. The head and neck would be one stone, the torso to his waist and wrists would be the second, and the bottom stone would be his legs and hands.

He would be a heroic figure, like a modern-day Kouros, inspired by the ancient Greeks and Egyptian tomb sculptures. In my mind's eye, his left leg and right arm would be striding slightly forward, his arms and hands held tightly to his sides. His right leg and left hand would be held back with hand fisted, while his head would be facing straight forward.

The sculpture would be nearly life-sized, standing on a hat rack with room for many hats. The idea was that it would find a permanent home in a children's facility such as a Ronald McDonald House. There, families and friends could donate a hat to the sculpture as a means to offer their own sick child a token of healing.

All compositional decisions were made to serve the metaphor of containment, as there was so much emotion to contain in this memorial. The sculpture would be quite stiff, its movement implied. The forms and proportions of the body would be fuller than in life, and there would be no folds in the clothing, further giving it a sense of intense inner pressure.

Each day that I worked on it, I lit a candle and did a meditation giving thanks for Sam's life. I would invite the highest purpose of this sculpture to unfold, so that it would be an instrument of healing for all those it would touch.

Usually, when I begin a sculpture of this sort, I first peg the stones together. However, I was so anxious to get his portrait visible that I left the pegging for later. Consequently, by the time I did peg the head, the fit was more challenging, as the stone had been rounded on top. The results were that the finished head is looking slightly to the right.

I WORK WITH stone as a two-way "conversation," a relation ship between the stone and me. As such, when something unexpected occurs, I respond to it not as an accident, but an opportunity brought about by the subconscious mind. I can either go with the flow or fight it. Whichever I decide, there is always a lesson to be learned, a new process on which to embark, or a message on offer.

I chose to see this change as perfect for the sculpture. The right side is often seen as that of the future, the conscious mind, the material world. So I allowed the change and moved forward with the sculpture, as its process had begun, predictably, to take on its own life.

Over the next few months, the middle and bottom stones were completed, with the exception of the right arm.

I took time out from the lower portions to complete details of the head before starting the right arm.

It was not until then that the process became wrenching. I had planned in my mind to have the right hand open at the very front of the stone with the thumb pointed forward. It was my intention that it be metaphor for Sam's life moving forward in spirit form.

As I completed carving the hand from the tip of the thumb backward, I stood away a distance for a broader view. I was horrified to see that the thumb was pointing straight down, the other fingers fisted, and that the stiffness of the right arm position made the whole arm and hand look dead. It looked so uncomfortable that I began to cry uncontrollably. How could I show this to his family? They had already suffered so much pain, and this arm would take their eyes *and* their hearts down into despair again. If *I* could not bear to look at it, how could anyone else?

The shock of the right arm frightened me not only personally but also professionally. I'd been teaching the figure for years and had never before created such visual discomfort. My earlier works were consistently calm visually, even when I was dealing with painful subject matter. I was surprised at myself at how insecure I felt to exhibit this work in an art community.

I could not look at it again for two whole weeks. I meditated on it and talked it over with a very wise friend who knows my work well. Over the years, I have learned not only to trust the creative process, but even to be guided by it. This sculpture felt like more of a challenge than had ever before been presented to me, and a new level of trust was a stretch of inner work that took some time to work through.

Instead of creating a memorial that simply honored a wonderful young boy's life, this work also described the horror of his loss. It was like two sculptures in one. Walking around it on the left side, I saw a playful little hero; but as I moved toward the right, my head bowed and my heart ached.

It was still, at this point, unclear how the juxtaposition of the forms would come together compositionally. However, I knew the sculpture was challenging me to let go of some preconceived ideas I held about myself as well as about Sam.

As it would happen, there was an exhibition coming at Christmastime, just a few weeks away. I felt strongly that it would be appropriate to show the sculpture, as it was to be an education-based show of artists who conduct workshops in local schools through Rutgers University. If this sculpture was to be included in the exhibition, time was short to complete it. Moving forward in the faith that the sculpture's purpose and resolution were being revealed to me in perfect timing, I mustered courage enough to face it again.

My plans were to include some gold and silver leaf on the surface of the stone. In past works I'd used gold and silver leaf as metaphor for precious objects and those that needed protection. I had carved a toy pickup truck on the overalls' chest pocket of the sculpture, and made plans to have this symbol embroidered on the caps I'd purchased for the sculpture. The carved toy truck, which was very dear to Sam, was to be solid gold leaf, as were the sneakers, which were images of his favorite pair. I sent the caps and the logo to a local embroidery shop with instructions for the truck shape to be filled in with gold stitching.

In the meantime, my very perceptive youngest daughter stopped by the house. When she saw the not-yet-painted sculpture, she began to cry and said she loved this sculpture more than any other I'd made. I described my plans for color and gold- and silver-leaf patination. Immediately she said, "You shouldn't use gold or silver on this one. It's not about you and your process anymore. This work is about Sam's life, and he was just a little kid. The sneakers should be just as he liked them—white."

I replied that the caps were already sent to be embroidered, but that I would consider her ideas seriously. I liked what she'd said about the work, but I was unclear how introducing white into the composition would work.

The next day, the hats were delivered to the house, fully embroidered. To my surprise, the truck logo was not a solid gold truck as ordered; instead, it was a simple but powerful white-outline drawing of the truck.

The universe had spoken again, and this time it was loud and clear! The means to finish the sculpture flashed in my mind's eye. Instead of gold and silver, the sneakers would be white, and the truck logo on the overalls would be a white outline on navy blue pants.

The sculpture's shirt was originally going to be a solid bright blue, as blue was Sam's favorite color. However, it became clear that by changing the shirt to wide horizontal white and blue stripes, the strong horizontal composition would compensate for the downward visual pull of the right arm and thumb, thereby incorporating all parts of the sculpture. Although the pain and despair of Sam's passing were still there, the horizontal lines around the upper torso visually contained it within the whole composition. The stripes invite the viewer to keep moving around the sculpture and not get stuck, visually *or* emotionally, in any one area.

With its hat rack now full of hats donated by people who knew and loved Sam, the sculpture stands as a testament to the pains and joys of caregiving while offering some comfort to those it has touched.

Members of Sam's family have expressed gratitude that the sculpture was created. His father described to me an emotional experience he had while spending time alone with it, and how its dual aspects both deeply affected him. Quite understandably, he chose to sit for a while on the left side of *Boy with Many Hats,* lovingly remembering Sam.

Let Me Tell You
What Happened . . .

∾

Barbara Sauvage

Let me tell you what happened with the man who
died that one night after I gave him the morphine. Sounds
like I killed him, doesn't it? That's what I thought. But I was
wrong. I need to think it out. I have chest pain just sitting
here writing. No chest pain when I walk fast, just when I sit
and think. I suppose someday I will think myself to death.

The man was 95. Parkinson's, very frail, wooden
response. But coherent. Just tired and slow, said his son was
coming, he was parking the car, would know what medications he was on.

He held a bucket of vomit with him, brown. I ran a
Hemoccult test, and of course it was positive. That means
bloody. His belly hurt, and he said he had been vomiting
since last night. We were in room 17, which was really 15, 16,

and 17 crammed together with curtains in between; a cart was up against the wall.

The son came in and said it started with the mother throwing up, and then the father. I put the man on the monitor, started an IV, called his doctor, told our doctor about it, and got some orders for Pepcid, I think, or Protonix. They did a CT scan of the man's belly, and his doctor came in and wrote orders for his admit, ironically enough not addressing the GI bleed—oh well. I can't remember what the admit diagnosis was now. Maybe abdominal pain. I found out later he had prostate cancer, that there was something on the CT that could have been a stomach mass, which could have been verified with clinical follow-up, had there been time for that.

I gave him the gut meds, and the son came out and said his dad was still in pain, so I called his doctor, who gave me an order for morphine, 1 milligram, that'd do the trick. As I said, I gave it. Then I went about the business of sticking my finger in the leaking dike that had become the ER. It was 6:00 P.M., or 1800 hours in military time. There had been no breaks for the nurses, and this was a 12-hour shift, or at least had started out as one.

About 15 minutes later the son came out, and stood there at the nurses' desk quietly waiting his turn while I redirected the psych patient who wanted to go out for a cigarette.

"When? When can I have a cigarette?"

"As soon as security is free. I'll get you a sandwich in the meantime, I promise. It'll be okay. Please go back to your room; I'll be there in a minute." Then I looked up at the son.

He said, "I'm sorry, you're busy, but could you come look at my father?" The son looked . . . confused.

I put my chart down and went into the room. The man was doing agonal breathing. Unresponsive. I stared at the man, not believing, I suppose, but trying to figure out what was happening and what to do about it. His son said, "He doesn't look good, does he?"

"No, he doesn't," I said, and added that I'd be right back. I grabbed Dr. M. and said, "You have to come into 17."

"I don't know the patient," he said, because of course we were holding patients in B and C, and the doc-before-him, who was gone, had done the admitting. So—*poof*—the man wasn't really in the ER anymore; he was admitted to the hospital.

He was just being housed in 17.

Dr. M. didn't have to touch him.

I said, "He's dying."

"Is he a Full Code?" Dr. M. wanted to know.

He was bargaining. Like Jesus at the wedding feast at Cana, he was telling me, *Woman, it's not my time.* But Dr. M.—a man who could tell you on any given day what saint's feast it was—knew where my head was at and that I would not let him go.

"He's a DNR," I said, pleading, shortening the command not to revive. "But the family is in there and they're going to want something done. . . ."

So we went back. I got respiratory from bed 16 to call someone down, and a nurse came in and we bagged him, although she had to do it because I grabbed the pediatric bag. The son was there; Dr. M. stood close to him, calm. They talked, decided to give epinephrine, atropine, and of course Narcan, so that the guy could really feel what was going on—the chest compressions, for example, when his heart went down to 39—but no intubation. *Gotta draw the line somewhere. Jesus, it's so messy; it's never anything but messy.* There was no right way to do this. There was nothing right about this.

His blood pressure went up to 170/110, heart rate 90; he was breathing on his own, it was a busy ER, there was nothing else to do, it was the end of shift, it was time for me to go home, 7:30 P.M., or 1930 military time. I really really really wanted to get the hell out of there.

But I stayed with the man and his son for two reasons. First, it was the right thing to do. Second, I didn't want the son to think I had killed his father.

This made me ashamed. But I thought, as I often had, in my crazy Irish Catholic skull, that just because you have an insincere motive doesn't mean you don't do the right thing. Suck it up and hate yourself, but do the right thing.

Sometimes I chose not to do the right thing because I was punishing myself: "Why are you doing the right thing, to make yourself feel better?" They call that scruples, whatever that means. I stopped not doing the right thing because it made me feel better when I stopped believing in God. Or sort of stopped believing in God, the Irish Catholic version at least. So I stayed, and hated myself for staying. I actually thought I had made this all happen with the morphine. One fricking milligram of morphine.

So of course the son asked, "Was it the morphine?"

"No," I said, trying to swim to the surface of truth even though I was busy torturing myself by thinking, *It was the morphine.*

But it wasn't, and I laid it out so he could see what happened. I laid it out slowly, because I owed it to this man who wanted to know why his father was dying, suddenly dying: "If it was the morphine, he would have revived with the Narcan. It's been my experience that people who are dying sometimes relax into it when they receive pain relief. It's not the morphine. Your father came in vomiting blood; there was something going on inside."

I understood while I was talking that the reason I wanted this man to believe this, aside from the fact that it was true, was that I did not want to be blamed for what was happening. But even though I did not want to be blamed, and even though I was ashamed for not wanting to be blamed, I told the truth.

I got Dr. M. to order a dopamine drip when the man's pressure went to 60 systolic. It was futile, but the son's wife was coming, and it wasn't time for the man to go, if I could help it. He did regain consciousness, and he squeezed his son's hand, and the son and daughter-in-law told him they loved him, and he mouthed the same to them, and then that was enough time. I took him to the unit so that he could finally be in a room by himself with his family, so that he could lie on a bed that wasn't a cart behind a curtain in a madhouse.

When I got back to the ER, we got a trauma case. A 40-year-old who went through the windshield of his car. I stayed. Because it was the last night I'd be working with S., who had the sense to go into obstetrics at another hospital, and she was as distraught as a charge nurse in ER hell could be. There was a guy at triage pretending to have chest pain so that he'd be seen sooner; there were people on carts in the halls, squads coming in back-to-back, a woman at the desk screaming that her cousin had had back pain all week and we better get back there *now* with some meds, a drunk patient fighting with security and the boy nurses in the Quiet Room, and another big red-eyed woman at the desk wondering when the hell she was going to be seen for her vaginal discharge, she had been in the room for 45 minutes and nobody'd come in yet. . . .

And we had Dr. P., the ER night doc who was recently moved from a city hospital because he couldn't cut it there. He wasn't cutting it any better here, but that was our problem now.

Also, and to be truthful, I was doing penance, or at least trying to get the taste of the old man's dying out of my mouth.

I actually forgot about it until 11:30 P.M., or 2330 military time, when his family came through the ER on their way home, because he was dead. I hugged them and told them they had taken good care of their father.

The hard part, said the son, was going home and telling the man's wife that he had died. They had been married 64 years; the man who had died had told me that, and I had made some joke about how he'd better be keeping his wedding ring on in the hospital.

"When are you here till?" asked H., a tech in her first year of nursing school.

"Seven thirty," I said. It was 1:00 A.M., or 0100 military time.

"You're a team player," she said.

"Or just nuts," I said.

I overheard J., who was taking her prerequisites for nursing and worked in the office but came out to play unit secretary when they really wanted to torture us, talking to H. about H.'s plans to work as an ER nurse: "So you want to be a trauma mama?" She was so pleased with herself for using this phrase, although I am quite certain she did not make it up. I was so pleased with myself for not choking her. At any rate, because they were short a nurse and there was nobody to call in, I volunteered to go on the run to Level 1 with the motor vehicle accident (MVA), which is what the gentleman who forgot to put on his seatbelt would be called for the duration. I promptly rescinded my offer when he came back from CT with news of a spleen, a bleed, a C1 fracture, and a systolic pressure of 70. That's why God made helicopters. And besides, one guy dying on you per night is my limit.

I went over to help lift in surgery, where they had just taken out his spleen—it was in a bucket they passed around to us ER folks. I looked at him and thought, *What if this was K.?* The nurse anesthetist was fixated on trying to get the guy's scissored jacket out from under him. He said he thought about those guys who'd come in, dressed up for a night out, nice clothes, maybe on their way to the tittie bar, and then they come in here, and it's all over. I wondered why a man on his way to the tittie bar would have a wife and son weeping at his bedside, but it was way too late to try to make sense of that. I finally got to leave at 3:00 A.M., or 0300 military time, and at 5:00, birds chirping, I crawled into bed next to K., who was not on a slab intubated.

It took me two days to tell him about it. I walked around quiet for 48 hours and then I asked him if I could tell him what happened that one night, and I sobbed and he listened and talked sense into me, because I had left my sense in the laundry room next to my blood-flecked shoes.

The Good We Do

~

Anne Caston, LPN

To loosen, a little, the girdle
in which death had cinched a man I knew,
I left my midnight charting and stole from the
    nurses' station.
Nothing strange in that, nothing
anyone would question.

Everything about my long walk down that
    darkened hall
seemed right and, at the same time, wrong.
Sterile walls shone in the half-light; fresh
wax gleamed and squealed under my soles.
On the door to the man's room

tonight, a new sign: *No CPR.*
Well, then.
So be it.

I stepped past the sleeping wife.
Such things are easy enough to do.
I turned the oxygen off and loosed the mask
that had strapped him to the flow.
Beside the bed, a Gomco gurgled noisily.

He gurgled too in the sludge of lungs gone bad.
I shook him; he startled, and would've cried out,
but I held the forbidden thing close enough
that he could make out what it was
in the dulled streetlight from the window.

I placed it on the bedside tray.
Back in five, I whispered, and stepped outside
to wait. I didn't want to watch.

It's strange, don't you think, how the good we do
we do loudly. But our sins?
Those we ease into in secret, and quietly.
And quietly was how I waited in that dim hallway.
Not for five, but for ten full minutes.

I eased back past the woman who was bruised
        with exhaustion
and watching over him. I thought he too had
        drifted off.
But when I turned to leave, he sat up, took my
        hands in his,
and blessed me, hard, for what I'd done.
        My hands
stung from the fervor of his blessing.

He rested well that night
and died some days
later, as we'd expected.

One cigarette. It was the singular kindness
    I could give,
though even that was wrong. I know that;
    I knew it then.
But the needle he'd begged for—"to end the pain"—
I couldn't give him that. Not that. Not
coward that I was.

I tell you this today, not to confess, not to
clear my conscience. I say it so it's clear to you
I believe I might be living yet
because of the furious blessing
he bequeathed to me that night.

I say it so you'll know
how it is that I have come to live
deeply in the shadow of my own guilt

and an old misplaced sense of mercy
which—despite anything
I might have once told you otherwise—
has at its center for me still
an odd, fierce comfort.

PART THREE

Reincarnation

*Informed commitment that
arises after sustained trail*

Why I Like Dead People

~

Sallie Tisdale, RN, BSN, OCN

Maud is 86 years old and weighs just that many pounds. She is nearly bald; her thin, fine white-gray hair has been rubbed nearly away by all her years in bed. At her age she is balding around her genitals as well, worn and loose where the catheter tube emerges. She is bare like a young girl, but the work of decades has left its erosion.

Maud had a stroke several years ago, and then another, and another. She doesn't open her eyes, never speaks. She is fed with a big plastic syringe that the nurses slip past her resisting lips; the right amount of pureed chicken or spinach tickles the back of her tongue and makes her swallow, involuntarily.

Tonight I discover that Maud has cellulitis, an odd but common infection under the skin. Her right hip and buttock are red, swollen, hot; she has a temperature of 104 degrees. I call her doctor. He asks me, "If you were her granddaughter, would *you* want me to treat her?"

"I'm not her granddaughter," I answer.

"You know," he sighs, alone in his office, wanting to go home, "I promised that lady years ago that I wouldn't keep her alive like this." He pauses, and I wait. "I *promised* her." Eventually he orders an antibiotic, because of the slight chance Maud's infection could spread to another patient, and her temperature drops in the evening, and she goes on.

I AM OFTEN asked how I can stand my work, and I know that it is this very going on that my questioners mean. Not only the uninitiated, but other nurses and physicians often dislike this "gutter work" that I do: part-time charge nurse in an old, not very good, urban nursing home, working with the sickest patients, the ones who won't recover from an unfortunate age. Some of the nurses I work with are always looking for a "better" job, competing with the thousands of other nurses for the hospital positions grown suddenly scarce in recent years—hospital jobs where patients come and go, quickly, and sometimes get well.

I feel a measure of peace here, a sense of belonging that is rare for me anywhere else. Partly it is because I know what to do, because I am competent here. Over the years, though, the ease that I've felt since my first job as a nurse's aide when I was 18 has become layered with fondness, the way one grows used to a house and its little quirks, the slightly warped kitchen floor, the sighing upstairs window. Here, all is aslant, and I have to tilt my head a bit to see it clearly.

Coming to begin a shift, I pass the activity room, crowded with humpbacked, white-haired people asleep in wheelchairs, facing a man playing "The Star-Spangled Banner" on a musical saw. In the corner, one upright, perfectly bald man spins slowly around and around in his chair, like a windup doll, bumping the wall at last and spinning back the other way. This is a scene of astonishing absurdity, and no one is paying any attention to it. We take it for granted, like the faint, lingering smell of urine tinged with kitchen steam and disinfectant. I leave the elevator on the third floor and step into furnace heat—July without air-conditioning—and the queer conversation of the confused that will dog my steps all evening long. They give me this gift of skewed perspective like a gift of non-Euclidean sight, so that I become as willing to dip and bend with the motion of a damaged cortex as a tree in the wind. I pass medicine room to room, and in each room the television is tuned to the same channel. For my four o'clock pass, it is *People's Court,* plaintiff and defendant, as I travel down the hall. As six we watch *Jeopardy!* "It's the only military medal that can be given to noncombatants," says the host, in Monte's room; then I pass Sylvia next door, and together we guess: "The Medal of Honor." And we are right. Bent over a task, preoccupied, I am startled by the peculiar speech of the nerve-worn, its sudden clarity. Up here, each day is the same, a refrain, and nothing can be taken for granted, nothing.

I know how many people hate nursing homes—hate the word, the notion, the possibility. A friend of mine lives next door to a local nursing home, and she tells me she hears people screaming in the evening, their voices leaping the tall fence between. She assumes the worst, my friend: that they scream from neglect, from abuse, from terror. She says it is a "terrible place," never having been inside. (I am similarly fearful around big machinery, in boiler rooms and factories. I am out of place, adrift, and fear the worst: Is that shower of sparks routine, or does it signal disaster? What is that loud noise?) I tell her that in every nursing home, there are people who scream, that they scream without warning, at private phantoms. I ask her where such people should go; I ask her how she would stop them from screaming. She listens, and I know she is unconvinced. Nursing homes are terrible places, she says, and it is because what happens there is terrible.

I enjoy my work, but I enjoy it in moments that are separated from each other by long stretches of fatigue and concentration. I enjoy it best when it's over. I catch myself, hot and worn at the end of the day, hoping the man I keep expecting to die will live until the next shift. I get irritable, and the clock creeps past 11:30, past midnight, and I'm still sitting with my feet propped up, trying to decipher my scribbled notes. The undone tasks, the unexplained events that want explaining, badger and chafe. And everybody dies.

My ideals twitch on occasion, like a dog's leg in a dream. I want no one to lie in urine a moment; I want every ice pitcher filled at every moment. For many years, I disliked the use of sedatives and antipsychotics to knock out the wound-up chatter of restless, disoriented souls. The orders read: "PRN agitation"—as necessary—and this is the nurse's power to ignore, and the power to mute. So easy is misuse, so simple. But just as a shot of morphine can break the spiraling cycle of pain, so can a spiral of panic be broken—not for my comfort, but for the comfort of the panicked.

Sadie screams at me from far down the hall: "Help! It's an emergency!" And she screams over and over, rocking back and forth, till I come to see; she leans over and points at the blazing fire under her bed, a fire she sees and hears and smells, raging out of control. I see no fire. I coo to her, hushing; she babbles on. Finally I lie beside her on her bed; she is stiff and yearns to leap up. And, at last, I go to prepare the syringe: "From the doctor," I tell her, because Sadie loves her medicine, and she falls asleep.

The responsibility is mine, the consequences are mine. I have to be sure about choices no one can be sure about. I call for nurse's aides to come and hold the flailing arms and legs of Charlie, more than six feet tall, furious at the world that confounds him so. He squirms and tries to bite me when I hit his hip with the needle. We all fall across the bed together, grunting. And I know that the visitor, passing by, sees only the force, the convenience, the terrible thing we have done to this person: the abduction.

The same is true of the smell, just barely there, acrid in the heat. It's true of the drooling, the patter of nonsense in the dining room. Visitors tremble, knowing Grandma is here, and wish they had the courage to bring her home, out of this awful place.

COULD THIS INADVERTENT audience, my patients' families, see these scenes and believe me when I say it is a labor of love? Some do; they bake blueberry pastries and bring doughnuts for the nurses, pat us on the arm, cluck their tongues. "I don't know how you can stand it," the niece said, after an afternoon at Aunt Louise's bedside.

The difference here is in what we each call love, the gap between their definition and mine. Their burden—and they seem to really want to know—is a burden of despair, a personal burden, bred of fear and impotence in equal amounts. This personal despair imagines as its opposite, its anima, a personal love and a personal sorrow. The visitor sees May defecating helplessly on the rug before anyone can stop her, and it strikes his identity, his self. It is as though the observer himself stood there, revealed. I have the advantage of knowing May will forget it in an hour; he does not. In breathless confession, waiting for the elevator, the visitor says, "I pray to God I die before this happens to me." I am told this again and again: "I pray to God." A kind of ego-terror is born, and with unbordered empathy comes flight. Suddenly the sounds and smells oppress, overwhelm. Suddenly it's time, more than time, to go.

A labor of love, love for fading people who dwell in shadows. I am saved from the need for flight—I am uninjured—because I let them do their own suffering. This is a cold-sounding excuse, I know. Call it compassion instead of love. (I am surprised, and pleased, just now, to find that *Roget's Thesaurus* lists as a synonym for *compassion* the less lofty *disinterestedness*.) I have learned not to make personal what I see. Just as the witness imagines himself, complete, transported to this place and trapped, so does he grant full awareness to those who are. He assumes Maud is aware of her plight, ruminates on her fate. I grant Maud plenty, without granting full cognizance to her withered brain. Down the hall from Maud is a man in his forties, paralyzed from polio, limited to a respirator, and he *is* fully cognizant: no pity for him, either. Pity makes distance, creates a separation of witness and participant; by assuming a person is absorbed in suffering, the witness prohibits him or her from participation in anything else.

I close the curtains, keep my voice down, as a point of etiquette as much as sympathy. I have a spring in my step; I can see and hear; I can eat and digest and control my urine, and I know these for the blessings they are. I am young enough, still, to take care of the old. But these are the most transient of graces, these graces of health, and I might lose them all tomorrow if the brakes fail. Old and sick comes later—but it comes.

Here, everybody dies. We tell black jokes. (I laugh and laugh at a cartoon of an old man sitting up in bed, surrounded by impatient doctors: "These are my last words," the old man says. "No, *these* are my last words. No, no, wait . . . .") We have a three-part mythos of death here, and first is that no one dies when we think they will, always later. Second, if a person long ill and silent suddenly comes to life, he or she will die soon. And last, people die in threes. Within a day or week of one death will follow two more. Just last week, Monte died, days after we'd predicted, and now Mr. H. down the hall is talking again, after months of sleep.

Death is anticipated, waited on in suspense. It is like waiting in a very long line that snakes around a corner so you can't see the end. When the last breath is drawn, it is startling; here is a breath, and another, and another. Death is the breath after the last one. Always fresh, always solemn, and not unlike a childbirth: the living let their own held breaths go, and smile, and in the solemnity is an affirmation. Here it is. I stroke the skin so suddenly and mysteriously waxen. I pull out tubes and patch holes. I like dead bodies: at no other time am I so aware of my own animation. This isn't because I am lucky and this poor fool is not, but because here before me is the mute, incontrovertible evidence. Some force drives these shells, and it drives me still. I am a witness, an attestant, to a forsworn truth.

Still I have my own despair. For me it is the things undone that break my back sometimes, the harried rush with people calling, and all those unexplained events. I wish we could ferret out the meaning in all this chaos, talk it out. No time—sometimes the ice pitchers are dry all night. Last week I had a shift like this, split in the middle by an impatient doctor who snapped his fingers at me and tapped his toe in frustration at my slowness. An hour later another doctor dropped by, and I asked her to see a new patient with a minor but uncomfortable problem. She refused, and then explained. "Medicine is the kind of job where you have to be really careful not to let people take advantage of you," she said. "Somebody always wants something." And all I could do was look at her, and get back to work.

I have to remember to temper my criticism of the aides, who work at least as hard as I do in a job of numbing repetition and labor. Hardest to remember, when so much is left unfinished, is what I have managed to do. I think I've been of no help at all, and then I realize how little help I'd be if I got discouraged and quit. Every task, no matter how late, every kind word, no matter how brief, makes a difference.

In my first job as an aide, I cared for a Swedish woman named Florence, who had only one leg. She was happy and confused and didn't know she'd lost her limb. Time and again she would try to walk and fall. I tied her in her chair, in her bed, and over and over she managed to untie herself and fall, thud, to the hard tile floor. She was always surprised. Exasperated at least, I stood over her and asked, "What am I going to *do* with you?" And she looked up from where she sprawled and said, "Don't stop trying, dear."

Don't stop trying. This is far from the best nursing home. It isn't the worst. I rant, jump to complain, go home frustrated. It should be better. But the sheets are changed, people are fed, for the most part each one is treated with kindness—a clumsy, patronizing kindness at times, but many of them don't discriminate on these fine points. Kindness is enough. Thousands, no, hundreds of thousands of people have joined these ranks, saved. There is no place to go but on, and on.

I like dead people and all their apprenticed fellows like Maud, who, slowly, is learning to die. And I like this place, with its cockeyed logic. I will feed Maud her squirts of puree, and a few minutes later Sadie will announce she is the queen of Germany and requires royal treatment. Celia will cough up blood, and, as I consider my options, I will hear the distant bed rails shake, the curses, the rhythmic, pattering singsong. Sometime the borders shift even further. I sprawl across a bed, fiddling with Roberta's leaking catheter, trying to disentangle her fingers from my hair. The feeding tube drips on my leg. Who is keeper, who is kept? This is the Marx Brothers all grown up, slapstick matured, life imitating art imitating life. Down the hall the Greek chorus begins, explaining the meaning and the mystery as the melodramatic story limps along.

Addendum

I wrote this essay in my second year of nursing. That was 24 years ago, and it is remarkable to me what has changed and what has stayed the same in the world I describe here. The long-term care of the fragile elderly and adults with dementia and chronic mental illness remains one of the most difficult jobs in nursing. But a quarter-century later, this is still an unappreciated and underpaid part of nursing, and largely in the control of for-profit corporations. The brief surplus of nurses I allude to in the story has become an acute and growing nursing shortage.

For quite a while, I stopped nursing to write full-time. I returned six years ago, to acute oncology care. Recently I returned to palliative nursing and the care of this vulnerable population. Much has improved, especially the emergence of "memory care" and "secure care" units where people can live safely on their own terms, largely free of physical and chemical restraints. Many of my clients are like those in the story, but now they are living in foster homes with families or pacing in safely fenced gardens. They die naturally, comfortably, and are not forgotten.

The Safe Zone

~

Anne Webster, RN

It's like when you were ten, and your mother calls
and calls for you to come in from a game of tag just
as the lightning bugs begin to flash, and her voice
gets that sawtooth edge you know means trouble.
It's when you run inside and flop down on the couch.
After she's done fussing and the crease between
her brows erases, she undoes your stubby braids,
pulling her fingers through your hair, a tingle
like dancing fairies that makes your eyes fall shut.

Or it's like that trip to Prague, all night knotted
in a plane seat, an hour of riding over bumpy roads
with a driver who doesn't know a word of English
as you hug your bag with money and passport,
knowing that if you disappeared now, no one
could find you. It's after you pay the driver the sum

he writes on a slip of paper, even if it's too much,
so he will hand you the key. When you lock the door
and your head hits the pillow, the dreams start
while your eyes are still open, and you can let go
of the thick meringue pressing on your brain.

Except this time you're curled in a hospital bed,
the air-conditioning on your backside, the only air
moving, certainly not in your lungs, that festering
mucous swamp, and you pant like a hound in July.
You don't dare sleep: sloppy nurses could bring
germs to finish you off or flood your heart with
the IV's two-step drip, the blood's thick crawl.
It's this new nurse, just when you've given up.
It's her stare over a stethoscope as she nods in time
to your stuttering pulse, reads the news in your
lungs' wet paper wheeze. At last you can rest,
your lids drooping like sheets hung out in the rain.

Redwoods

~

Laurie Barkin, RN, MS

LAST NIGHT IN bed, thinking about what the day
would bring, I remembered being in a redwood forest—the
cool moisture on my face, the spongy brown duff of the
forest floor with its swaths of green sword ferns, a cathe-
dral of impossibly tall trees enshrouded in fog. And the
silence. Lush and comforting. It's no wonder Jean-Michel,
our neighbor and friend, wanted to die in Guerneville under
the redwoods.

Although he made a living as a master cabinet maker
in the city, Jean-Michel poured his passion into the cabin
he built in Guerneville, a gay enclave 90 minutes north of
our neighborhood in San Francisco. A few years ago, he
told Brian and me that he had just hung ten-foot-wide slid-
ing glass doors in his bedroom. "Now from my bed I have
a view of the redwood grove. You must come up sometime
with the children." He smiled as if he were already there.

"You know, redwoods are the tallest trees on earth, but they have shallow roots. So, to keep from falling over during storms, they weave their roots together. I love this about them—it is like they are holding hands underground!" I think this is how Jean-Michel felt in Guerneville, surrounded and supported by a community of friends who gathered there with him each weekend.

This morning we've decided that Baby Ben and I will represent the family at Jean-Michel's memorial service on Cemetery Hill—a ridge high above his cabin—leaving Brian on daddy duty for our older two kids. I had hoped for an earlier start, but after throwing in a load of laundry, scrambling eggs for my five-year-old daughter ("I only like the way you make them, Mommy"), and unshackling my screaming two-year-old son from my leg, Ben, our insatiable three-month-old, decided he was still hungry. For a second I had entertained the idea of driving up north by myself—but, no, I'm breastfeeding. Ben and I need each other for mutual relief and nurturing. So, after he has been nursed and burped, I change his diaper, load up the baby bag, and buckle him into his car seat.

Ben begins fussing shortly after we cross the Golden Gate Bridge. But at 70 miles an hour on 101 North through Marin County, I can do little to comfort him. A light sprinkle of rain soon turns into a steady stream that slows traffic. At the same time, Ben's fussiness escalates into angry wails. When we finally arrive in Guerneville an hour and a quarter later, too late to attend the service, Ben has fallen asleep, it's pouring, and my head aches. Instead of driving up to Cemetery Hill, I follow the directions to Jean-Michel's cabin. Other cars begin to arrive soon after I've parked. The service was probably cut short by the rain.

Although hunger will wake him up soon enough, Ben snoozes as only fat babies and old, overfed cats can. While doors slam and people run into the cabin, I take a few moments to calm myself. Raindrops drum the roof of the van like thousands of fingers tapping a desktop. Water flows over the windshield in a drapery of gray silk. In the dim light, my thoughts turn inward to the night just before Jean-Michel died, when I visited him at Davies Hospital.

Brian and I had a neighborly relationship with Jean-Michel — sharing seeds, plants, and even a few dinners — but we were more cordial than close. Although I am a nurse, when I visited him in the hospital I refrained from asking him questions that I would normally ask a terminal patient. Would you like to talk about what is happening to you? Have you spoken with your family? Do you feel at peace or in conflict? Is there someone I can call for you? Instead, I freshened his water, cleaned off his tray table, emptied and replaced his garbage bag, massaged his neck and shoulders, and rearranged his pillows — containing my feelings under an invisible nurse's cap, avoiding the intimacy of his dying.

As soon as I returned home from the hospital, I handed the car keys to Brian who took his turn visiting Jean-Michel. An hour later, he returned and trudged up the stairs. "Hold me," he said. We stood like that for a long time. Brian, an attorney, had never before sat with a dying person. "I felt so helpless," he said. "All I could do was hold his hand and pat his arm."

"That was the best thing you could do," I said, noting the irony that my husband, more intellectual than emotional, could feel so much about Jean-Michel's dying, whereas I felt muffled, out of sync, under water.

Maybe it has to do with my work as a psychiatric nurse consultant on a trauma unit. For the last three years, I've spent my days listening to story after story of freak accidents, falls, stabbings, shootings, and torture. I try to keep an open heart, to empathize and connect, but such terrible knowledge comes with a price: palpitations, paranoia, nightmares, and irritability. When those of us who do this work asked for time to talk about how we cope with what we hear, we were told that staff support groups are "not billable" and therefore not possible. My six-month maternity leave couldn't have come at a better time. Although I love my job, I am worried about its effect on me. Over the years, I've seen a few nurses turn their feelings off altogether. *Maybe it's already begun to happen to me.*

During a break in the rain, I unfasten Ben's car seat and transport him to the front door. Once inside, we pass through a vestibule hung with umbrellas and jackets before entering a living room filled with people. Large vases with dried flower arrangements anchor the ends of a long table covered in white linen and set with colorful platters of food. My neighbor, Philip, Jean-Michel's housemate, greets me at the entrance. "Let me show you a quiet place for the baby. Then I'll give you a tour."

Bypassing the living room, we enter the bedroom where, sure enough, the glass doors that Jean-Michel installed frame a stand of redwoods. Save for a chestnut brown leather chair and ottoman, a simple bed covered in dark blue, and a night table, the room is spare. In my mind's eye, I can see him relaxing in his chair with his feet up after a day of woodworking, gazing at the grove of redwoods and planning the next day's work. I place my sleeping baby on his bed and take advantage of the privacy to speak with Philip alone.

Philip tells me about Jean-Michel's last few hours; how they signed him out against medical advice, how Philip and Jean-Michel's other friends tried to keep him alert and comfortable during the journey, how they settled him down on a pile of blankets and pillows where he died minutes later looking up into his beloved redwoods. I hug him and tell him he did right by his friend.

Philip wipes his eyes. "Come, let me show you the kitchen," he says. Once there I can feel Jean-Michel's love of craftsmanship in every inch of the room. Philip, an architect and designer, points out the counters Jean-Michel fashioned from pink-hued hemlock, the armoire he made of oak, the cabinet handles he fashioned from madrone, and how the kitchen cabinetry matches the wood-paneled walls in the living room. I wish now that we had visited Jean-Michel here when he was healthy. I would have enjoyed seeing the pleasure he must have taken from showing off his work.

After making sure that Ben is still asleep, I sit on the couch with a plate of food and watch Jean-Michel's friends as they support each other through yet another loss. A few weeks ago, at Jean-Michel and Philip's annual Christmas party, I danced with some of them to Gloria Gaynor singing "I Will Survive!" Now they stand with their arms braided around each other, recounting tales of happier times. Mimicking Jean-

Michel's thick French Canadian accent, one man says, "Een New York, Jean Michel vuz zee toast of Zee Beeg Apple!" I'm sure it's true. Even when I first met him, before the ravages of AIDS, Jean-Michel was hunky and handsome.

Soon, my full breasts ache. With my ear to the bedroom door, I hear the beginning of Ben's hungry sounds. Seeing me, he wriggles and smiles a true smile, not the kind accompanied by gas. While he waits for my breast, his eyes light up and his tongue laps against his lips. Once we are situated on the leather chair, he wastes no time. "You greedy thing," I say, feeling the smooth squishiness of his supple body against mine. Ten minutes later when I unlatch him to switch breasts, he bristles. "How dare you!" he seems to say. After he burps, I resettle him and help him find the other nipple. "Yes! Yes!" his body responds. "I've found it again. The source of all happiness!" After burping up what seems to be most of the milk he sucked down, Ben rewards me with a dazzling smile that makes it all worthwhile. After a smooching session, I carry him into the living room.

"Could I hold the baby?" asks a sweet-faced man.

"At your own risk. He's a prodigious spitter-upper."

The man lays the cloth diaper over his shoulder and holds Ben to his chest, supporting his head with an expert's hand. Whispers of "baby" sweep around the room. When Ben burps up some more milk, the sweet-faced man calmly mops it up with the diaper. Others ask to hold him, and soon Ben is passed around the room like a ladle of water among people thirsting to remember that life gives as it takes away. Later, as the mourners leave, they thank me for bringing the baby. Although I didn't plan it this way, I too am glad.

With only a handful of people left in the house, I carry Ben back into Jean-Michel's bedroom, closing the door behind us. Once again we sit in the leather chair where I sing to him until his eyes close. Looking out to the redwood grove, I picture Jean-Michel laid out on the blankets smiling up through his beloved trees. Then, other faces appear: Alice, who gripped my hand though a difficult night on a ventilator; Jack, who died waiting for a heart transplant; Stuart, a schizophrenic boy who hanged himself behind his parents' home. When they leave, I feel a swelling in my chest. Tears begin to fall on the blanket I've wrapped around Ben's slumbering body.

It feels good to finally cry, but now I wonder: Will Ben absorb my sadness? Will the combination of crying and breastfeeding deplete me? *No, I don't think so.* Emotions are like a nursing mother's breasts: the more they are tapped, the more they replenish themselves.

On the way home I imagine Jean-Michel's community of friends—their arms braiding themselves into strong cord, weaving themselves into a fireman's net, a blanket, or perhaps a trampoline. This is what we need, those of us who open our hearts to our patients' traumas: a blanket for comfort, a fireman's net for safety, a trampoline for resilience. Maybe instead of standing like lone pines, we could become a grove of redwoods, our roots entwined, holding hands underground.

Slow Night in the ER

~

Anne Webster, RN

We've got a man with gas gangrene.
I look up from my crossword puzzle,
raise an eyebrow. Gas gangrene?
It's a couple of hick ambulance drivers
who've seen too many old movies.
But one of them is carrying a big carton
marked "O Positive," so I pay attention.
They drag in a stretcher, blood
dripping off the sides. *He was working*
under a truck, and the jack slipped.
Wheel rim caught his belly.

The patient, a black man, mid-thirties,
clutches at the sheet with callused hands
when I tug it down to see something

more personal than his pecker; ropy blue
intestines studded with brassy fat spill
onto the gurney. By then I'm on the horn,
calling for orders: stuff the guts back in,
cover the yawning wound with saline
soaked towels, pump in more blood.

I can't do it. My hands won't work.
I stand outside the curtain, shaking,
till his soft voice comes at me. "Miss?
Are you there?" I glove up, put on
a big smile, walk through those drapes
like a movie star on Oscar night,
"We're going to fix you up as good as new."
I keep up the stupid grin, lifting the dead
weight of hot guts as I feed them back
into his belly's maw. "How's the pain?"
I ask. "Just a little." He points to a tiny nick
on an eyelid. I think maybe there is a God
until a week later I hear kidney failure
killed him. Now I know not even
my winning smile could have saved him.

Visite d'Adieu

~

Diana Mott, RN

I IMAGINE IT STARTED something like this: I was sitting on a park bench, absentmindedly observing the parade of joggers, bicyclers, and dog walkers on the asphalt path that loosely followed the course of the Hudson River. The watery thoroughfare in front of me was dotted with sailboats and kayakers and the occasional Circle Line cruise boat, brimming with weekend tourists seeking a more romantic vista of the city. All around me, recreation took on its many forms, from the frenetically aerobic to the languidly inert; the *New York Times* remained unopened in my lap. My reverie was interrupted by the tinny bell-tone version of *Ode to Joy* that heralds my cell phone calls. It was my friend Cathy.

"I'm here with Annie. We are both depressed and trying to come up with something really great to do to cheer ourselves up. We're thinking Paris. You interested?"

"Sure," I answered, without blinking an eye or considering family obligations and the frightening exchange rate. Who needs money when she has a credit card? I am a pushover when it comes to travel under just about any circumstances, but an offer of a weekend in the City of Light with two women my age and no agenda but eating, drinking, and talking? This was irresistible. Within 24 hours, Lucy had been added to the party, and the following day we had plane and hotel reservations on hold: my potential travel companions were no-nonsense businesswomen who were accustomed to putting ideas into action with frightening efficiency.

As a result, I began to hesitate. So much money for a long weekend. Such short notice—we would be leaving in just two weeks.

"Annie is ready to book the flight, so you need to decide if you are really serious about going" was how Cathy interpreted my "Sure" from the day before. She was well acquainted with my tendency to procrastinate.

"Absolument!" I heard myself say. At that very moment, I realized that I *was* sure, because I loved Paris and wanted to wander around the Marais and go to the d'Orsay and eat foie gras and drink red wine and jog along the Seine, but most of all, I was sure because this trip would provide me with an opportunity to visit Vivienne.

Almost a year before, Vivienne had come into the oncology office where I work as a chemotherapy nurse. She was a renal pathologist in France and had come to New York for treatment for ovarian cancer and a fellowship position at New York–Cornell. A doctor I know told me much later that she was a world-renowned resource in renal pathology.

Vivienne would never aggrandize herself like that. I once asked her how she became interested in her specialty, and she said, "When I was a young mother, I needed to work part-time and found an opening with a pathologist. I discovered that I had a good memory for slides and could remember, in detail, a slide that I had seen weeks before. And I fell in love with the way cells look under the microscope."

A plain woman in her sixties with short gray hair, large teeth, and laughing blue eyes, Vivienne possessed a warmth and friendliness that made her keen intelligence all the more attractive. She was a famous doctor. I was an oncology nurse. Yet she sought my opinions about her symptoms and side effects and loved to share the small pleasures of her week. "I felt so well yesterday, I even cooked a chicken!" she would say as we walked to the infusion room. As she settled into one of the three lounge chairs, I would think of a medical issue that I found puzzling: "What are the risks of the testosterone injections my friend is taking to reduce aging?" I would inquire as I swabbed her skin where I would place the needle. She would delight in explaining things, and could be expansive but never patronizing. Her appointments were scheduled at the end of the day, when I had time to sit with her; over time, we got to know each other and conversed as friends do while the chemotherapy dripped into her veins. Partial responses to some of the treatments enabled her to work, go to concerts or visit friends, and, most memorably, enjoy her teenage grandchildren's first visit to New York City that Christmas. Ever the armchair tour guide, she got a kick out of their discovery of the city and talked animatedly about their visit long after they had gone back to Paris. In the spring she spent happy weekends walking on the beach and dining with friends on Shelter Island. By midsummer, she was no longer responding to chemotherapy. She decided to return to Paris to be close to her family.

I had said good-bye to Vivienne six weeks earlier, in the waiting room of the oncology office. It was an emotional leave-taking because I thought I would never see her again. Vivienne was sanguine; she took my hand in hers, gave it a gentle squeeze, and smiled as she said, "You must come to Paris and have a meal with me." And here I was!

ALTHOUGH EVERY FRANCOPHILE I talked to and every memory I could retrieve told me that the eighth arrondissement was the wrong (right) bank, Lucy had a connection at the Prince de Galles on boulevard George V. Our suite of rooms was luxurious, and so was the neighborhood: the swanky Champs-Élysées with views of the Eiffel Tower or the Arc de Triomphe, depending which way you turned your head. It was the neighborhood of Hediard, Armani, Louis Vuitton, and little French shops selling $500 cashmere scarves and €7 coffee crèmes. In our first hour at the Prince de Galles, while waiting for our rooms to be prepared, we ate omelets and drank coffee in the hotel restaurant. It cost $150.

After fully exploring the accommodations and declaring that I wanted to live in my immaculate white-tiled bathroom with gleaming fixtures, towel warming rack, and three-foot-deep bathtub, I made a phone call to Vivienne. All my plans for the next three days would be built around my anticipated visit with her and her husband, Gregory.

Vivienne and Gregory lived on boulevard Raspail in Montparnasse. The Metro directions were easy: *Take the green line from Charles de Gaulle Etoile to stop Raspail; walk down Raspail to number 257.* It was a lovely fall afternoon, and the residential neighborhood was quiet. I bought pink roses in the only place I could find, a tiny corner shop that specialized in funeral arrangements.

I thought she looked a little thinner, but she wore a merry smile and was genuinely happy to see me. We drank tea and sat in her small garden and talked, warmed by the early-afternoon sun. When it grew chilly, we moved to the high-ceilinged living room, where, surrounded by books and photos, Vivienne was clearly at home on the small couch. I imagined her holding court there when family and friends dropped by. Gregory said they even had occasional dinner parties in which Vivienne was an active participant. I was glad to hear that she had found a good doctor who respected her desire to be kept comfortable and to stay at home. She seemed content, perhaps even optimistic. Of course, she didn't think about food, and I became very hungry during the visit, especially when I remembered that my travel companions were at a favorite restaurant, eating foie gras and Brest chicken while I was in Montparnasse drinking herbal tea. I stayed too long because it was so hard to take my leave.

Finally, pulling the heavy wrought-iron gate closed behind me, I stepped onto the pavement. I decided to walk for a while in the last of the autumn light and soon found myself in the Jardin du Luxembourg. Here couples sat on metal garden chairs and read the newspaper or held hands while children played, and students congregated and smoked cigarettes and laughed, and families strolled under the espaliered pear trees. I stood at the low wrought-iron fence that surrounded the beehives, funny wooden boxes of varying heights with spindly legs and octagonal metal hats, lined up and looking like they would come alive and start to dance. Next to me, a young father was crouched beside his son, pointing through the fence stiles. A dog was barking. The park was full of life.

The Reason Nurses Write Mostly Poetry

∼

Kathryn Gahl, BSN, BS, RN

The reason nurses write
mostly poetry (as opposed
to screenplays, short stories,

or a novel where imaginary
people play pretend
and fool even themselves)

is because nurses revolve in systems,
each spin part of a process
diagrammed like a sentence

with tightly crafted schedules
for meds, change-of-shift reports, and
don't forget our homecare nurses

pumping out paperwork, the lactation
consultant pumping you know what,
and tired instructors with students

linking verbs and predicate nouns
into diagnoses, well, it's easy to see
how a nurse hurries to convert heart sounds

and hard words into art before the next patient
arrives, hemorrhaging, counting on that nurse
to flow like a pen, bleed for them both.

Notes on a
Nursing Home

~

Ann Neuser Lederer, RN, BSN

A FEW YEARS AGO, after a futile job hunt, I accepted
work as an aide in a nursing home, which I will call Mullens
House. I had recently completed a degree in anthropology
and somewhat naively looked forward to the aide experience
as an adventure.

Having never before entered a nursing home, I was
shocked by the encounter. A new world challenged my view
of reality. It haunted my dreams at night and eventually led
me to become a registered nurse.

I have since entered hospital nursing, but memories of
the nursing home cannot be suppressed. They call out not
to be hidden in some recess of the mind or soul, even as the
confused elderly are so often tucked away in the corners of
institutions.

It was an old persons' home, perhaps nicer than some. The odors, masked by disinfectant, were not overpowering as I stepped inside. And there was some sense of community—the residents were not only similarly aged and ill but also shared a tradition, a religion, and for many, friends, family, and memories. The administrators and staff took every opportunity to celebrate birthdays, anniversaries, and all holidays. And so, in the beginning, it seemed a not unhappy place.

The area I was sent to work in, I later discovered, was considered the most difficult unit. The back corridors, uncarpeted and stark, were reserved for the most confused residents or those unable to control their bladders or bowels or in need of constant supervision so they would not wander away.

As my defenses threatened to turn me away or to make the strangeness ordinary, I reminded myself: Be sensitive, open. Do no injustice to anyone's reality. Allow. Accept. Do not force or impose.

Wide, expressive eyes were everywhere, watching, mirroring. Soft voices murmured in various languages, reenacting ancient conversations. Rows of thin old people reached out toward any affection. The aides played Big Mama, as though caring for large infants. They hugged and scolded, changed diapers, and bathed.

A thin finger beckoned from across the room. In a small gruff voice a woman whispered, "How are you?" I was elated. For weeks I had thought she never spoke.

On a day off, I could do nothing but sleep. I dreamed often of them, and the old women spoke to me in voiceless whispers: "We sit in a circle and sing our songs to no one in particular. We have little to learn from each other's wisdom. We repeat the same chant in our separate voices, not hearing the chorus for our deafness: 'I am old, my husband is gone, and my children have their own lives. I am ready to die.'"

I answered their whispers with my eyes. "Let me take your arm, old woman, I'll step into your dream world. With your blurred eyes you see granddaughter, cousin, mother. 'Mama,' you call in a childlike voice, but then suddenly you say, 'Look, honey, I know you're not Mama, but what does it matter?'"

The rhythm band came to entertain. Social workers passed around toy xylophones and triangles. The old ones pounded on them or clapped or wailed. One couple got up to dance. "Let me call you sweetheart. . . ."

I did not ask the silent ones for their stories. They knew too much to tell. It was better to wait patiently for a glimpse, and then carefully piece together the grand tapestry. In the long hours of the nursing home, there was an illusion of endless time.

The memories still follow me, some flickering, some sharp and clear, like snapshots.

Papa runs through the hallway, feet bare, shouting, "The horses, I must feed the horses!"

"But, Papa," we say, "there are no horses here."

Subdued, he follows us back to his room. "That's right, they're in the stable." A large man, he towers above the women in white who order him about. Everyone calls him Papa, taking their cue from his wife, Mary.

It is rare for both partners to survive into their eighties, and those few living here are honored. Papa and Mary have separate rooms a few doors from each other, because she frequently disturbed his sleep by checking on him throughout the night.

As I wash Papa's face with a cool cloth, he is crying softly. "I feel sick. I'm so weak. If Mary isn't asleep, let her come to me."

Juanita allows no one in her room. When she came here, the aides say, she screamed as they took the kerchief from her head, revealing a mass of tangled hair and lice. Sometimes she reaches a haggard hand from the door of her room and hollers our names in a ragged voice. Some of us, in a hurry, try to walk by Juanita's room, ignoring her demands, knowing she is too lame to follow. If you pause, she pulls you close and makes a small request—a glass of prune juice, a cookie, a pill.

A party is held for residents born in July, and the social workers invite her to come.

"No. I ain't going. Big Eyes look at you. Big Eyes is the devil."

Juanita is afraid of the evil eye. She bangs about in her room, making her anger known, enjoying the attention she has brought on. After the party, her carnation and a large piece of cake are brought to her.

Mr. McElroy sits in his room after meals, preferring to be alone. He is a delicate little man with keen gray eyes, and silent most of the day. But sometimes he becomes a demon—biting, kicking, spitting. It may take four of us to get him out of bed. Behind his whiskers, he seems to be laughing at us.

Mabel is 102. Nearly blind, she holds her eyes tightly shut against all light. Her thin hands are fists that no one can pry open.

Each morning the aides comb her long, snowy hair and roll it into a little knot, adorned with a red ribbon. She seems scarcely aware of these ministrations. But when they bring her tray, she cries out, "Feed me! Feed me. Oh, Mommy, that tastes good." They spoon the pureed food into her tiny mouth.

Once, I saw Mabel sitting naked on the toilet, a bedsheet tied under her arms and around the handrail to keep her from slipping off. A group of children moved through the corridor, singing holiday songs. Her door was quickly shut as they approached, but she hummed the Christmas carols along with the children outside.

Ms. Cottle is up at dawn. All day she sits in the lobby, watching with one eye the TV programs she has chosen. Her other eye is on the flies, two or three on the window, one on the floor. Once in a while she hops up to whack at them, without success. Finally, in the middle of the national news, she kills one.

"It stole my blood last night," she claims, then smacks the carcass again, just to make sure. She seems satisfied with her revenge.

You would think they'd been married their whole lives, the way Lucy scolds George and the way it quiets him. But this is a second marriage for both, and has lasted only a decade. He is now 95, "an ill-tempered devil," his wife says.

Though deaf and nearly blind, he still manages to pinch the aides as they go by.

Lucy and George were found half starved, his legs gangrenous, their mattress full of money, and they were cajoled into this home, where they share the same room. He must be lifted from wheelchair to bed now that his legs are amputated. Lucy leaves their room to watch TV or play cards with the other women when she's sure he is comfortably settled.

Rebecca lies wheezing, alone. Wordlessly, she waits in the quiet room, inviting death. She refuses to eat, shaking her head firmly at all food and pills. Her only adornment is a gold wedding band and her black, shining eyes. She is so beautiful, it is heartbreaking to watch her grow thinner by the day. The nurses insist that she must be gotten up, must be bathed daily, and fed.

When I help Rebecca to the tub, she clings tightly around my waist as she walks, facing me, in a macabre dance. After her bath I hug her close, dripping wet. She says nothing.

Each day I fill a large syringe and try to squeeze the protein and vitamin solution into the corner of her mouth, but her jaws are clamped shut, not to be pried open by those who would have her live.

Gertrude asks, "Where is my home? I want to see my grandmama."

I say, "Think, Gertrude. You are not a young woman. How old are you? Eighty? Ninety? Do you think your grandma is still alive?"

"No, and I'll soon be dead too."

"Then maybe you will see your grandmother."

"No. You die, you go under the ground."

Ed shuffles down the corridors, his face in a wry grin. He stops to smile and say in the loud voice of the very deaf, "My son took my watch back with him to the city to be fixed. You know, to be without a watch is like eternity—time goes around and around. It's endless."

When Ed's son visited, he tested his 82-year-old father's mental ability by giving him numbers to add or subtract, and questioning him about current events. "The old boy's still pretty sharp," he said proudly, before returning to his distant home.

Not long after, we heard a loud bang from Ed's room. While climbing to hang an alarm made of coat hangers above his door, he'd fallen and broken his left hip. One of the more confused women frequently wandered into the wrong bedroom at night, so Ed had decided to be warned of her arrival.

After his fracture, he spent weeks in the hospital, and when he returned his mind was not the same. Now he is strapped to a chair to prevent him from wandering, and given a television and crayons to occupy him. With the crayons, he writes on the TV and table, "Help me!"

When I first approached this foreign world, I was frightened by the twisted faces and disjointed speech. Gradually I saw it as a separate world with its own structure and rules, its distinct classes.

Among the residents, the elite were those who were still in command of themselves. The ones who were confused, who had to depend on staff for their most basic needs, were the underclass.

They were not mistreated or neglected. More nurses and aides were assigned to them than to the elite. They were just marked as separate: by their living quarters in a special wing, off the beaten path, where visitors and others need not be reminded of their presence; by their uncarpeted dining room; by their incontinence garments; and by their eyes—sad, hopeless, wild, or simply blank.

Marked as separate too by being taken once a week in a long train of wheelchairs to a special room where they were reminded of the day, the month, and the name of the president. There they were given little heaps of sugar and salt to taste, then asked to tell what the tastes were called.

The confused were marked too by being placed at night on a layer of blue absorbent pads and restrained lest they crawl out of bed and wander away.

Even the staff mirrored these distinctions. Those looking after the elite scorned as hard and dirty labor the work of the others. The aides caring for the underclass said they could not tolerate the petty demands of the elite or being treated like servants.

These aides often acted like mothers to the helpless residents, protecting them from stares and comments. Before any were to be seen by outsiders, the aides carefully cleaned and dressed them in their best. They were perfumed, the diapers and catheters concealed with robes, old slippers replaced with shoes. Sometimes an aide would apply lipstick and rouge to each woman.

But the aides could also be stern and often raised their voices in anger. "Look at her filthy fingernails. She's wet again! Someone get the mop. Somebody comb her hair."

Small wonder that so many of these old people lay awake at night, watching the light change to darkness outside the window, calling for Mother, or singing old songs as lullabies to help bring sleep.

I worried that I would become too accustomed to this world, that I would, in time, become insensitive. Some of the more experienced staff advised me to will that change. "Don't let what you see here get to you. Don't think about it when you go home. Don't fall in love with any of them."

I watched others who had been submerged in this world as they argued or ridiculed. I resolved to remember the larger context—that these residents were vibrant individuals, frantic for their last expression of independence. Petty demands and obsessive rituals were ways to guard one's territory in that insistently communal place.

Although tempted, I tried not to act as a mother. Many had had so much done for them for so long that they seemed to expect being treated like children: "What shall I do now? What dress shall I put on?" I tried not to encourage this behavior and thus speed the loss of their independence.

It takes much less time to dress a slow, disoriented old man than to let him do it. It is more efficient to feed fumbling old people than to wait and then clean up the mess afterward. But soon they have forgotten these skills.

Who is to blame for what they have become? Do we segregate them so we need not see and be reminded that their fate may one day be ours?

Perhaps it is the very healthcare "system" that crowds so many into these places but offers low incentives, in pay and social recognition, to attract caregivers. Those who do come are usually not previously trained, as I was not, in caring for the old, and certainly not for the demented. It is exhausting work. The body aches at the end of the day, and the spirit is soon broken from so much sadness.

In a recurring dream I walk into a room, reach out to touch a thin, papery arm. I move my fingers down to the hand, feeling the knotted veins. Quickly, hand grasps hand and clings tight. The eyes do not seem to see, yet the hand holds with the strength of centuries.

Slowly, from the depths of the spirit come ruminations. "I too was once young. . . . Now I am—look at me—tired . . . old."

Even the very oldest cling to the belief that they are persons, strong in their individuality, and not part of this grouping, this world of confusion.

How do we respond to them? How should we respond?

Night Shift

~

Mark H. Clarke, RN, BSN

I am a nurse who works at night
taking care of your father
who is dying.

I work at night taking care of your dying father
who can't sleep;
what's the point, when so much sleep lies just ahead?

Your dying father can't sleep
and I'm his nurse,
so we sit up in the night talking.

He talks of you in the dying night
when he can't sleep
and I must stay awake tending to him.

He tells me of the pride he feels for you
and the joy he feels at the sight of you.
There, in the dark,
he doesn't bring up the things you retain:
the shaming words,
the fiery temper you feared to face.

In his dying night
he doesn't mention love either,
perhaps out of his own shame
for the murky residues
he knows he left in his love for you.

If he seems especially sad about the interminable night,
and I feel strong enough to bear it,
I tell him I'm a father too,
and I trust my children will somehow feel my love,
whatever memories they may retain.

After helping him to his feet and holding him steady
so he won't have to urinate lying in his dying bed,
so he won't have to urinate lying in bed like a baby,
he says: "You're a good man, Mark. . . .
You remind me of my son."

The Swim Lesson

~

Laurie Barkin, RN, MS

AFTER MY KIDS walk-run to the far end of the indoor pool, just in time for their lessons, I settle into a yellow plastic chair in the viewing area, eager for a half hour of peace. Even though it's exactly 8:00 P.M., this is the first moment I've had to myself all day. In my work as a psychiatric nurse consultant, I tend to absorb my patients' pain like a sponge. So each week here at Baby Baleen Swim School, I arrive eager for the time and space to wring myself dry.

In my rush to make dinner and get the kids to class, I had forgotten to change my clothes. Worsted wool pants and acrylic sweaters work just fine in the cool Bay Area air but cling and itch in this jungle-like humidity. My hair, barely tameable in the best of circumstances, frizzes. The smell of chlorine seeps into my head and I start to feel irritable again, the way I feel each day at work when patients we've barely patched up on the trauma unit, where I spend most of my time, are discharged to the harsh glint of the street. Mismanaged care, we call it.

To calm myself, I take a few deep breaths, but soon I hear a child crying. He appears to be about four, lean torso still longer than his legs. Shaggy black hair obscures his eyes. Except for a smattering of freckles across his nose and cheeks, he looks Asian. His father (I assume), an imposing man with reddish hair and the same smattering of freckles, delivers the boy to Sabrina, the swim teacher, who waits for him at the shallow corner of the pool closest to where we parents sit.

"Kenji, stay with Sabrina," he commands. Before his father turns to leave, Kenji lunges for his pants. "Nooooo," he wails. Dad releases the boy's fists, turns him around, and pushes him toward Sabrina, who opens her arms. "Come with me, Kenji. We're going to have fun." Kenji trudges toward her, chin on chest. After a few steps, he stops and looks back at his father, who has taken a seat in the plastic chair next to mine.

"Come sit here with me, Kenji," says Sabrina, whose smile could land her a toothpaste commercial. Kenji takes baby steps until he comes within arm's length of Sabrina and the two other children in the class. Then he sits down and pulls his knees to his chin like a pill bug, curled into himself.

My kids—older and long past tears—are stationed at the opposite end of the large indoor pool, where I can barely see them. Throughout the 30-minute classes, I look in their direction at regular intervals and wave when they see me. That way, they'll never suspect the truth: although I look like an attentive parent, I'm really zoned out in a galaxy far, far away. Usually, that is. Today, I give my full attention to the father who carries himself like a marine drill sergeant and the kid who looks as crushable as an insect underfoot.

At least Kenji's dad is here. Among the patients I evaluated today—most of them young men with gunshot wounds—one dad was killed by the police years before, one is in prison, and two long ago abandoned their families. Although absent, these dads are very much present in the stories their sons tell me, young men with big holes in their hearts in addition to the ones caused by bullets. *My kids are so lucky.* Brian works long hours, but when he's home, he spends his free time playing with the boys.

The swim teacher, Sabrina—mid-twenties, big and blond and wise to the ways of children—allows Kenji to remain on the deck while she fits the other two kids in the class with goggles and flippers. Kenji remains curled into himself even as she takes him in her arms and follows the two girls as they wiggle and giggle across the width of the pool.

Maybe the noise and the activity overwhelm him. At any one time, seven classes line the length of the pool. Shouts and whistles bounce off tile and concrete and echo through the cavernous space. Kenji reminds me of a patient who kept a sheet drawn over his face for days, refusing to allow the outside world in. Maybe Kenji is like that, easily overwhelmed by the noise and commotion of life, slow to trust, and wary of change. Or maybe it's just the psych nurse in me trying to figure him out.

In the pool, Sabrina swings Kenji around to her back. He clings to her like a baby monkey, his face buried in the nape of her neck. "Hold tight with your arms, Kenji, but let your legs float." When she releases his legs from her waist and breaststrokes behind the girls with blue kickboards, Kenji lifts his head up for the first time. He keeps it up even when the girls' legs spray water onto his face.

"Hey, that's progress!" I say to the dad.

"Mmm," he responds. Then he pulls out a newspaper from a black briefcase and snaps it open to the sports page.

Was I wrong to comment? I feel upset until I notice his right leg jiggling up and down with such intensity that my own chair vibrates. Clearly, this man has something else on his mind.

I know I should be watching my own kids' lessons. During the ride home they will grill me with questions to see if I was paying attention to them or if I was lost in my own world. This time it's neither.

When they reach the other side, Sabrina unhinges Kenji's hands from around her neck and seats him on the underwater steps. "Kenji, would you like to try flippers?" Her large blue eyes search his face for an opening. Kenji steals a glance at the flippers and frowns. Sabrina regards him for a moment, then sits alongside him. She places her hands in the flippers, stretches out her arms, and pretends she's a duck, paddling and quacking in a pond. In response, Kenji's lips curl up ever so slightly. Once I heard a psychiatrist describe doing the same maneuver when he interviewed a paranoid schizophrenic patient. "Moving along side him instead of sitting opposite him was the only way we could share something in common," he explained, "even if all we could share was the same view out of the same window."

Sabrina points one flipper at the girls and quacks, "Let's do that." Kenji shakes his head no but does not protest when she slips the black flippers on his feet.

The dad startles me when he jumps out of his chair, pulls his cell phone from his back pocket, and walks toward a dark hallway. Kenji tracks his dad's path until the hallway swallows him whole. A shadow of disappointment crosses Kenji's face. *Abandonment. Maybe a little abandonment this time, but lots of little ones can add up to something big.*

Stepping backward, Sabrina pulls Kenji toward her. Despite himself, Kenji kicks his legs. In the middle of the pool, when Sabrina lets go, Kenji dog-paddles to the other side. This time, delight illuminates his face. Kenji has discovered the magic of flippers. *Did his father really miss this moment?*

Suddenly I remember my own children at the far end of the pool. No doubt they've been trying to get my attention. As I search for them, the words of an elderly Greek patient come to mind: *When you point your finger at someone, three fingers point back at you.* The younger one sees me and waves. I smile and wave back.

Directly in front of me, Sabrina fastens Kenji's hands to a kickboard. "Let's see if you can get yourself all the way back to the stairs," she says. For a few moments, Kenji frowns, his recent success forgotten. In the meantime, Dad returns to his seat beside me. He clears his throat and hunches down, elbows on knees, head bent. He rubs his face and runs his hands through his auburn hair, sighing deeply. Now I'm irritated. I want to tell this man to step outside of himself and focus on his child, to offer him some encouragement the way Sabrina does. When Kenji motors himself back to the stairs, his father doesn't seem to notice.

It's late, and all of the other classes have ended. Kids swarm the showers. Sabrina collects flippers and motions Kenji and the girls to stand on the deck mid-pool, where the water is deepest. She picks up a red hula hoop and holds it high in the air. The girls scream as they jump like tigers through a ring of fire. Kenji sits down and covers his eyes. His father sits up and folds his arms across his chest. I hear his breaths, shallow and too fast.

"Nerve-racking, isn't it?" I say.

"Huh? Oh, I guess I wasn't paying attention."

That's an understatement.

After the girls jump a few more times, Sabrina sends them to the showers. Kenji is now the last child on the deck.

Suddenly, my kids are standing in front of me dripping wet. "Mom! Did you see me do backstroke?" says the older one. "Hey, I did it too!" says the younger one. "And I picked up all the rings faster than you did!" I squeeze a globule of shampoo on each head and send them to the showers, thankful that their one-upmanship got me off the hook.

Sabrina whispers to Kenji. Then she slips back into the pool, emerging a couple of yards from him. "How about here?" Kenji shakes his head. When Sabrina repositions herself in Kenji's comfort zone, he scoots over to the edge of the pool. He stands, then sits and returns to pill-bug mode. Kenji's father sighs and shakes his head.

"Oh well," I say, "there's always next week. I bet he'll do it then." I notice that my chair has started to vibrate again.

After shampooing and rinsing off, my kids head for the locker room. I gather my things and liberate myself from the plastic chair, which falls over and crashes on the concrete floor. "Sorry!" I say to the few parents still seated around me. Before I can right the chair, one of them points at the pool and cries, "Look!" I turn around in time to see Kenji jump into Sabrina's arms. Kenji's dad rises and strides over to the pool's edge, waiting for Kenji to climb out.

My pulse quickens. I fear that this dad will be too harsh on his small bug of a boy. And if he is, what will I do? Even if I could take him aside while Kenji gets dressed, how can I, a stranger, remind him that children remember everything—feeling helpless, frightened, abandoned, invisible, or inadequate—and that these memories make them who they are?

Kenji struggles to pull himself out of the pool. When his father does not offer a helping hand, my chest tightens. Once on the deck, Kenji stands in front of his father and lowers his head. I ready myself to intervene, not knowing exactly what I will do but knowing I will need to do something. Then Kenji looks up at his dad and smiles, not a wide Chiclet smile, but a shy, pursed-mouth smile. Dad bundles him into a huge beach towel and hoists him up to his chest. They cling to each other long past the time for a congratulatory hug, oblivious to the wet and dripping children who scuttle behind them.

I feel both relieved and confused. In the hospital, I try hard not judge my patients. I know that their addictions reflect histories of untreated trauma and rotten luck. I understand that poverty and neglect and infirmity bring out the worst in people. But here, as a parent, I've been less than charitable, quick to judge and, apparently, to misjudge. Lots of things could explain the father's earlier behavior. Maybe he was reliving a near drowning. Maybe he just lost his job, or maybe his wife is ill. I shudder to think how easily I filled in the blanks with scenarios from my patients' stories about absent or abusive fathers and how riled up it got me.

But none of it matters now. Before retrieving my kids from the locker room, I press the image of Kenji and his dad bundled together into a page of memory. Tomorrow, when I listen to the grief of grown-up children with holes in their hearts, I will conjure up this scene and smile.

Reflection

~

Marilou Carrera

Quick glance—
There was a photo—
I saw myself, I thought,
For just a moment;
There was the hair and the smile,
With the dimples and the wrinkles
In the corners of the eyes. That was me!
Had I been studying for hours on end
That day?
Or recovering from a night of well-earned play?
Was that the day I inserted my first Foley,
Maybe saw a cardiac catheter insertion,
Instead?
Probably I was laughing about the sleep
I never got,

Tossing and turning those nights before clinical.
Wasn't I fighting back tears earlier that day,
For a young boy who got Christmas gifts,
Three times over from the hospital elves?
No, I'm sure that photo was taken
Just last week:
After living those moments again and again,
I could still smile.
That is me.

Why I Stay

~

Katherine Suzanne Harris,
BSN, BA, RN

"How come you get to leave early?" one of the nurses demanded suspiciously. "It's busy; I want to go home, too." It was my first year as a nurse and I was working nights in a big hospital. Becky, a fellow nurse, was signing out a bit early, 5:30 A.M. instead of 7:30 A.M.

Becky replied, "Well, I'm sick; I've got the flu. I've been throwing up since midnight, but I had to stay until my patient delivered. There was no one else to take her."

Incredulous, I asked, "You've been throwing up all night, but you couldn't leave?"

Becky sighed. "Not until I finished my paperwork." She turned and walked down the hall. Everyone else carried on as if that were normal, while I stood there, my jaw dropped open. Now that I've been a nurse for seven years, I know nurses bear the brunt of poor staffing like this time and again.

There are plenty of practical reasons I stay at my job as a nurse. Believe me, I often recite them to myself when I'm overwhelmed and overworked on the labor and delivery floor where I have worked part-time for the last four years. Here's why I stay: I get paid $25 an hour (only $1 more than when I started eight years ago!), which is certainly not enough for the stress, responsibility, and wear and tear on the body, mind, and soul, but it is double or triple what I earned doing childcare or working in a health-food store, so I'll take it. My job also provides me with flexible hours, so I can switch off daycare with my husband, which has been wonderful for my growing family. Another big reason to stay at my job is my really amazing fellow nurses, who inspire me with their goodness and stamina week after week. They treat our patients with such love and respect, walking tirelessly up and down the hall days and nights, and they motivate me to keep working as a nurse. Of course, some aren't so good or inspiring, but after being on my floor a few years, I have established a place in the jungle and I don't get too much backstabbing from the nasty nurses anymore. And, I remind myself, I really do enjoy taking care of families and their babies. It is such an honor to be with people at such a sacred, transformative time. I know I'm lucky to witness babies coming into this world every week, even though I'm working hard; it is a blessing to be there and support women through such an amazing experience as childbirth.

This conversation I have with myself about staying at my job is frequent because even though I work in a pretty nice place, the staffing can be terrible, dinner breaks are a luxury, and I keep getting those pleading phone calls to come in on my day off. At least once a week we evening nurses have to draw straws at midnight to see who will stay extra because there has been a sick call or because it's busy and someone has to cover it.

Recently I realized another reason I stay at my job is that I am actually good at it. After seven years of working as a nurse, I have a reservoir of hard-earned knowledge and experience-based instinct that allows me to take good care of patients, ask the right questions, and demand help when I need it. It took a lot of hard work to get here.

Last week a first-year nursing student came to observe my fellow nurses and me at work; she sat shyly in the corner and stared. I could only vaguely remember how lost she must have been feeling—witnessing, but not getting, the understanding upon understanding that comes only after time. We were talking about a breastfeeding problem: "Her nipples are big, but the baby's handling that okay, I think he just hasn't figured out suck/swallow." Judy did an imitation of the baby's suck. "He's doing this: *smack smack smack*." We all laughed and knew just what she meant. Judy continued, "I did tongue exercises with him, and that seemed to help. We're using a cup with pumped milk. He's young; hopefully he'll figure it out before she gives up. I gave her a long pep talk today to try to keep her spirits up."

Seeing us through her eyes, I was floored by how much we knew, how many assessment techniques we had, the language we had developed to express things—and I was impressed. As a momentary outsider, I could see how much important specialized knowledge we had and how very lucky the patients, midwives, and doctors were to have us. Later the student said, "I can't imagine knowing all you know, all that you take for granted." I just nodded my head and said, "It takes time and really hard work."

Another reason I stay is that whenever I get sick, I am taken care of by nurses and realize how profoundly important we are. It happened again this year. At eight weeks of pregnancy I couldn't stop throwing up; my stomach muscles hurt from heaving ten times a day. I hadn't had food or drink for two days, so after I fessed up, my midwife sent me to the hospital. I stumbled onto the unit where I work, but as a patient this time.

Ellie, my fellow nurse, met me with a gentle guiding hand on my arm and brought me down the hall to a room with darkened lights and an IV pole ready. I descended onto the cool sheets and lay on my side while she started my IV with complete ease and got fluid running in my veins, asked my admission questions with quiet professionalism, reassured me that I would feel better after getting some rest. Then she left me to sleep soundly for four hours. When my parents came in to visit, my head kept lolling back as I fell into sleep while talking to them. They thought I had been drugged, but I hadn't. I could let go because someone else, my nurses, were watching over me.

I had been trying to eat but vomiting, trying to drink but vomiting, worrying and trying to take care of my three-year-old, while getting sicker and sicker. Once I was in Ellie's hands, I didn't have to do anything anymore.

During my four-day stay and two subsequent admissions, I was awed by my fellow nurses, how they assessed my condition, how they advocated for me with humor, grace, and frustration (when midwives were too busy or the pharmacy was slow getting meds). The nurses were the backbone of my stay. They witnessed my illness, my frailty, and gave me hope I would survive. There was something in the graceful way they cared for me that seemed natural and easy. I knew, because I was a nurse, that they were frazzled and had too much to do, but as a patient I never would have known it. They took the time to sit with me, to make my bed, to help me into the shower as I got weaker. Nurses don't get credit for much of what they do because it is so basic, so fundamental, but that is also what makes it so pivotal.

Barb would cock her head and ask, "How are you doing, Katherine?" and she meant it, really meant it. Healing is found in all the technical things nurses do, but it can't be denied that being listened to is healing, being understood is healing. Having someone who doesn't walk away when you start to heave into the pink bucket for the millionth time, tears of effort streaming down your cheeks, is healing. They were unafraid, they did not judge, and they did what they could to make me better.

When I went home, I continued receiving nursing care from visiting nurses. They came to my home, made friends with my dog, sat on my couch, and listened to my daughter chat about *The Wizard of Oz*. They assessed me, my IV, my medications, and my situation with comfort and grace. They kept me afloat in fluids; they were supportive and funny. I looked forward to their coming and felt like I had a net, a web of people supporting me and guiding me back to wellness; most of the web was made up of nurses. As I lay there in bed, I thought of how important my job is and how lucky I am to get to do it. Of course, there are many changes I hope to see, but the foundation of the job is dear to me, is second nature, and every time I get a whiff of it from the other side, I realize that it is a huge responsibility and wonderful honor.

In Honor of the First Anniversary of Your Death

~

Lise Kunkel

For my nontheist Quaker father

Like Socrates, you took the cup quietly—
though without a god,
and with a religion.

We helped nature take its course;
and now that your dying is done,
the lens pulls back for the living—
our focus again inclusive
of the neglected, the less than vital.
I would not want to live each day as my last—
a popular notion lately.

In each of my days,
I gladly nurture the influence
of your ordinary living:

an eye for the newly forming bud,
the progress of the violets,
which birds are back, which have flown,
the swell in the creek, food on the table,
a reasonably good red, a satisfying book,
a dedicated sense of fairness—a kindness

not always apparent in nature.

Coming Home to Nursing (Without Having Really Left)

~

Kathleen Walsh Spencer,
MSN, MA, RN, CS, CPSN

As a child, I was the little kid who always wanted to play school, happy to be the student or the teacher. While growing up, I couldn't decide whether to become an English teacher and writer or become a nurse. In 1974, when I graduated from high school, the economy in Detroit was very depressed. I chose nursing for the job security.

Once in nursing school, I realized nurses are teachers! After graduating from nursing school, I took a job on a surgical floor at a 1,000-bed hospital in Michigan. It was a huge adjustment to give up the student life and be responsible for patients' lives. I remember a patient asking me, "Are you old enough to do this procedure?" I had the license in my pocket but no experience.

The first September that I was working instead of going back to college, I mourned the college life. By January, I was enrolled in the master of science in nursing program at Wayne State University with the goal of teaching nursing. After graduation, I stayed on at the university to teach medical-surgical nursing. I felt it was important to have clinical credibility for my students, so I always worked weekends in the ICU. The faculty salary was very low, and I couldn't continue teaching and meet my main financial goal of home ownership, so I left after three years.

I took a clinical nurse specialist (CNS) job at a 350-bed hospital and covered all of the medical-surgical units. It took me several months to realize that trying to cover such a large area was setting myself up for failure. I carved out a niche as a wound care and ostomy specialist because there was a tremendous need. After three years at this hospital, I went "home" to be a CNS on the same surgical floor where I had been a general nurse.

My CNS role on this 72-bed unit had been a very happy and successful time for me. I already had good relationships since I already knew many of those people, so I didn't have to spend much time gaining trust and respect of the staff. I think the CNS role was one of the best jobs I ever had. The components of the CNS role—educator, researcher, consultant, and practitioner—offered me the variety that I craved. I love patient care and teaching. The research was interesting, and I discovered I had a knack for writing up research and clinical articles for publication. Presenting at conferences was a highlight of the role. I took the Dale Carnegie course in public speaking and was soon adding motivational speeches to my repertoire. I traveled throughout the United States and Canada to present seminars on clinical and professional topics.

The CNS role was a launching pad. I had a great group of colleagues, since there was a CNS on each nursing unit. As a group, we were really dynamic. I wouldn't hesitate to take that job back again.

During my time as a CNS, I went back to school again, this time in journalism. It was not because I was dissatisfied with nursing; it's just that I wanted to be able to do more for nurses. In the 1980s, the image of the professional nurse was suffering, largely due to media portrayals on television. There was a particular show, *The Nightingales,* by Aaron Spelling, that depicted busty nursing students as jiggling bubbleheads. I was on a mission to improve the media images of nurses, and I was going to do this by becoming a journalist myself to promote more positive media images. I began working on my master of arts in journalism through Michigan State University, one class at a time. The best part of taking classes was that I was in a mix of people totally different from me. I hadn't realized until then how narrow-minded I was about the world. I knew nursing, but not enough about everything else. I didn't even own a television! It was very rewarding to go to class at night and have these "media people" learn about our profession through me.

I was halfway finished with the program before one of the faculty suggested that it was time that I apply to it.

(I never did write the admission essay. Don't tell.) I wrote two papers in graduate school that I got to present many times across the country. One was "The Image of Plastic Surgery in Comic Strips," and the other was my master's thesis, "A Content Analysis of the Image of the Nurse on Get Well Greeting Cards." I realized how my words could reach others and leave a positive image for nursing.

I wasn't really looking for a job when I noticed a job posting for director of an employee wellness program. I had some experience as a consultant for the wellness portion of the Ford Motor Company retirement program, so I thought, "I can do this job," and interviewed for it. I didn't get it, but the interviewer said, "You'd be a great candidate for this other job that will be posted," and told me about the role of the internal communications coordinator (ICC).

This position would be brand new to the hospital, and they wanted a person who could hit the ground running. Whereas the hospital had a public relations department that handled communications with the world outside the hospital, the ICC would be responsible for all of the communications inside the hospital. This included producing the employee newspaper, running the management meetings, and doing whatever else the ICC could dream up to improve communications within the hospital.

I knew a nurse would be perfect for this job. We are born communicators, and we know the hospital environment well because we interact with all of the clinical departments and many of the nonclinical ones. We are by nature teachers and creative problem solvers. We understand patients—the reason the hospital exists.

It took a full six months to go through the interview process (there were 25 candidates) and another six months before I was offered the job. Why the delay? I learned later that top administrators weren't sure about the idea of having a nurse in that position. I still can't imagine what the downside would be, but they actually consulted a PR guru from the East Coast, and he was supportive of the idea. When I finally met him he said, "Nurses are good thinkers."

The day I started the new job, I picked up my new ID badge. *Administration* was written in dark letters across the bottom. I quickly realized that I was being treated differently. The people who served me in the cafeteria line, checked my books out at the library, or drove the shuttle bus didn't treat me the same as they had before; they were on their best behavior. You know the feeling you get when you walk into a room, and all of a sudden the room goes quiet? It was like that all the time.

More troublesome was the reaction from my nursing colleagues. Some felt that I had abandoned nursing, for bigger and better things. This was reinforced by the fact that my badge no longer had a big black *RN* printed on it under my name. Within a few days, I was back at the security office getting the *RN* added to my badge. I was just as proud of being a registered nurse as ever, and it hurt me that people considered that I was "leaving" nursing, when all I intended to do was use my nursing to influence patient care from a different perspective.

The job was tough. There seemed to be a question looming in the air if this position "would fly." My boss didn't let me put nail holes or hang shelves in my office. I wasn't given a computer, or access to the email system. The secretaries in the executive suite didn't support me, even in the small things. For example, my first Christmas season in the suite, they hung a wreath on every executive's door but mine. (My wreath was hung on the bathroom door.) One said to me, "We don't think a woman should be in this position." I gave myself pep talks. I would envision the Whac-a-Mole game at an arcade; the one where you clobber the mole with a big rubber mallet every time he sticks his head out of the hole. Too often, when a woman rises head and shoulders above the crowd, someone is always there with the big mallet. They beat me just because I was doing a good job.

One of the first activities I did was do an assessment of the current state of communications at the hospital. I interviewed a large sample of the middle managers. I was disheartened to realize that most of them thought I was a spy for administration.

I introduced a communications plan to the administrators, and the plan took a year to approve. I found that the administrator I reported to was known as a micromanager, slow to make decisions. In nursing, there had been more willingness to try new things to benefit patients, because the patient was lying in the bed *now*.

With the goal of improving communications top-down and bottom-up, I put a number of communication conduits into place: a monthly video newsletter, a newspaper for managers to share with their staff, a number of face-to-face communication programs for employees and administrators. Although I proposed about 15 new programs, only a few were implemented each year, one at a time. I feel great satisfaction that now, 12 years after I have left that job, all of the programs I had proposed have since been approved and implemented. In administration, I did not have the feeling of going home every day knowing that I had made a difference in someone's life.

It was the first time I was in a high-profile position, instead of being just one of several thousand nurses. Any missteps I made were obvious. Yet I had the authority to communicate my ideas to administrators, set agendas, and shine a spotlight on issues important to me, such as how insulting it is for a professional nurse to punch a clock (a system that was changed).

I found that in my role as the ICC, the employees were equivalent to my patients. I felt responsible for creating a good communication environment for them and wanted to keep them informed. I thought they deserved clear, direct, honest communication. In any organization, however, not every message can be communicated to the employees: we never outright lied to the employees, but there were times that we couldn't be as straightforward as I would have liked. This was troublesome to me.

Over the three years that I was the ICC and away from bedside nursing, I felt pangs of jealousy when the nurses would talk about patients on the units. The CNS group was still dynamic, and I missed being a part of it. Sometimes in a meeting I would look at my watch and think about what the CNSs would be doing at that moment.

The pressures of the job were growing: politics, problems with my employees (and little support from my boss), and very long hours (14 hours a day). I was tired, stressed, newly married, and having trouble getting pregnant. It seemed that the negatives of the job were outweighing the positives.

I had met with the director of human resources several times over the last few months in my job. I was looking for career advice. Was it possible to leave this position without damaging my résumé? Would this employee problem ever get better?

Some of my favorite administrators were those who still identified themselves as nurses. (I was surprised by the number of top administrators who kept it a secret that they used to be nurses.) One of these great nurses was the hospital director, who oversaw the department of anesthesia. I had confided my desire to return to nursing, and she was enthusiastic. "Come work for me!" she said, taking me by the arm and touring me around all of her areas. She clearly loved being a nurse, and that was exhilarating for me.

When I finally made my resignation known, the human resources director encouraged me to go through the proper channels. I met with the nurse recruiter. She said that I wasn't qualified for any nursing jobs since I had been out of nursing for so long (three years)! "I would rather take a GN than you, because their nursing skills are more current," she said. I was flabbergasted. How could she negate my previous 12 years of nursing experience? She had me fill out a transfer form for all of the open positions, but she said it didn't sound promising. I related this incident back to the hospital director, who asked, "Why didn't you just go through me?" One thing that had disheartened me when I was in administration was the lack of kindness and collegueship between the women, but I didn't expect this from the nurse recruiter.

I was terrified the day I cleaned out my beautiful mahogany office in the administration building. I took the paintings off the wall, packed up my files and photographs, and tucked away the Cross pen set that the staff nurses had given me when I got the job on administration row. I was sure that I made a mistake, but my replacement had been hired. There was no going back.

My reentry into nursing was uncomfortable. As I moved my nursing things (new clinic shoes, stethoscope, lab coat) into my locker, I was suddenly aware that I was on a much shorter leash. I was told when to go to break, when to go to lunch. Those first several weeks, I never got to eat in the half hour allotted because invariably I would be stopped in the cafeteria by an administrator or employee who wanted to talk. One day on orientation, I was a few minutes late coming back from a break, and one of the nurses made a huge scene in front of my peers. I had the feeling that I was a target for a lot of employees' frustrations with administration. Even though I was back in nursing, some considered me "one of them" and hurled complaints at me.

After a few weeks, I heard a rumor that I had been fired. The sentiment regarding my resignation as ICC was: "Why would anyone step down from a job like that?" Ouch.

I was surprised that it took me a full year of full-time work to feel comfortable with all aspects of clinical nursing in post-anesthesia care, which was a new specialty for me. The patients I was caring for included the plastic and reconstructive surgery patients, whom I always enjoyed. The care of plastic surgery patients was a common thread throughout my career. Prior to leaving nursing, I was a CNS for five years, and even though that is a clinical position, it is not the same as working directly at the bedside with a patient assignment, which requires a different set of organizational skills. It took me so long to get up to speed that I swore I'd never leave nursing again.

I think it is important for nurses to keep stretching themselves by taking on different roles, serving on various committees, teaching, publishing, or doing whatever is of interest. I had been writing columns for the Patient Education Department for *Plastic Surgical Nursing,* and was promoted to associate editor. In 2004, I became editor-in-chief. These positions were the perfect opportunity for me to blend my nursing and journalism skills, and I got to know nurses from all over the country.

Although there are plenty of days that I missed my administrative job, I am very happy that I came back to nursing. Each day when I go home, I know that I made a difference in someone's life, that his or her patient experience was better because I showed up.

Some days I do get frustrated about this career. If I think about it too long, I can really get irked by the fact that young people graduating with degrees in business and engineering come out of college and immediately start making double what I do after 30 years of nursing! Doesn't anybody see how important our jobs are? Nurses are far too undervalued. Still, I work as a nurse because I can't imagine not being a nurse. With the worsening of the nursing shortage, who will take care of the patients?

My other calling is poetry, which feeds my nursing self, and vice versa. I work out a lot of the heartaches in life, many seen as a nurse, through the healing act of writing poems. Poetry allows me to write truthfully about the emotions of being a nurse. Sharing these poems with non-nurses gives them a glimpse of how difficult and rewarding our lives really are. It is an honor to be a nurse and share the most intimate moments of a patient's life. Writing it down helps me savor this.

I want to keep my nursing license active as long as I can, and in Michigan, that means staying in clinical practice. I have been a nurse longer than I have not been a nurse. Nursing is as much a part of me as my birth order and signature. I am now in my 50th year, and it seems appropriate that I am examining what my career has meant. God willing, I will be able to practice as long as I want.

Without Permission

~

Carissa Swiatek

My instructor told us
we were not to do vaginal exams
and yet when my preceptor asked
if I'd like to follow her
I nodded yes
and slipped my fingers in,
shy in those strange fluids,
the opening already large
and frightening,
foreign and yet familiar
like sitting down
to afternoon tea in a new country:
the flesh warm,
the insides sticky, plush, deep.
I did not know what I was getting at,

what I'd gotten into exactly,
but I had an inkling
and I had to follow it home—
for this question
was unanswered
at the birth,
startling and blue and frank
as it was,
unanswered as mother and father
cooed and petted and wondered—
too fast it all seemed to happen,
too perfect and complete to witness
and yet I peered and felt
and will coax
again and again
out of my own greed,
disbelief, and unknowing,
aware I will never come to know
all the secrets within,
knowing that,
yet wanting to know.

Slate Blue

~

Piaf Latham-Wintergreen

I AM A NURSING student. I have been for some time. I have one great fear (well, in this case anyway), and that is changing an adult diaper. This is because I gag, uncontrollably that is, at really bad smells. So it terrifies me because I do not want to gag in front of a patient. I couldn't bear the incongruity.

Horrible.

So here I am, and I dread and I dread. Quietly, inconsistently. I usually work on the mother/baby, labor/delivery unit, which has its perks and its jerks, I suppose. Then yesterday, I was scheduled for a 12-hour and got floated to another floor. I was sent to sit with a patient. See, patients get sitters when they are on suicide precautions or fall precautions usually. It's a big legality. So, they pay me X dollars an hour to sit there and read and help people to the bathroom, change sheets, give them their trays. A long 12 hours, to say the least. That is why I always bring a book to work.

I walked into his room, his eyes piercing slate blue, sunken. The nurse had whispered just before I entered, "HIV, AIDS. Wash your hands. Wear gloves." I said what I always say: "Hello, I am your student nurse for the day; my name is P." I looked into that slate and smiled as I shook his hand. I wasn't wearing a glove. He was so handsome and regal with all four bed rails up, diaper on, and nasal cannula inserted. He wore his pride, and I respected him with all my might in that first moment. Patients often aren't treated like people in hospitals, as you well know. And I, sure as fuck, wasn't going to treat him like a nothingness death number.

I had the privilege of sitting with this man who is in so much pain he cannot get out of bed and who likes to hang one leg off the bed to touch the ground, for groundedness, until the nurses pull him back up in bed because they don't get the need to touch the ground when you lie in bed all day feet touching nothing but sheets that shear your heels. I washed his entire body, I slathered him with his special Kiehl's lotion, I powdered and I primped. I handed him his Gucci sailor hat, and he was happy. We listened to French mambo and Nina Simone. We talked about glass and memory and Paris. He offered to will money for my student loans. I told him his family deserves it more. He squeezed my hand when they drew blood, and he tried to hide his dirty diaper from me every time to preserve a sense of dignity. I said, "It's okay, I am not looking, I just want to clean you up so you can be comfortable." I gagged, quietly, when his back was turned. Thank goodness his back was turned. I am so sorry for you, my friend. I would change a thousand diapers for you. A thousand.

A Nurse Reads
A Book of Luminous Things

~

Elizabeth Tibbetts, RN

She picks it up in stray moments,
one poem while the water boils,
but on duty the book stays in her bag,
hidden and reassuring as her working heart.

At the moment, the towel dispenser
enrages her as it emits one inadequate
square of rough paper—seconds she doesn't
have—there are pills to give,

catheters and dressings to change,
and Mabel is sitting in her doorway crying forever,
"I'm so afraid, where am I?"
because the line from her mind to her throat

is broken, and touch, hot coffee,
a shawl, and Xanax haven't helped.
Outside the open windows, evening
is a lavender light and the scent of lilacs,

summer rising from earth's body,
the air ripe and shimmering.
Inside, the call bells ring,
a sound that pierces like a needle along a hem.

"Jesus," the nurse says quietly, unable
to imagine past 11:15, when she'll leave.
Up the hallway comes Joe in his wheelchair,
his feet walking as he wheels, lost inside

Alzheimer's incessant motion.
He pauses at the desk,
holds up a calendar for her, and says,
clearly, loudly, "June!"

and smiles so fully she can see the letters
click into place in his brain,
where the word is opening a road
lined with trees bent beneath the weight

of purple blossoms, and he is driving slowly,
the radio on, and his true love,
who's a very young woman, sits neatly
beside him when anything is possible.

I'm Staying

~

Shirley Stephenson, RN, MA, MFA

In a cold climate, respiration clouds the shiny horizon. Different lengths and weights of wire hang from the wall like rods in a bait-and-tackle shop. There are paddles, just in case. Two men wear camouflage kilts, tops and neck guards made of lead. They've got The Killers on the stereo: "Smile Like You Mean It." As if ice fishing, they drop a line into the body of water, Señor L., sedated but conscious in his twilight, a ruby puncture in his femoral artery. He can still respond and breathe profoundly. He can still trap air as the X-ray machine dips and rotates around him, an awkward serpent measuring prey. This is a routine morning in the cardiac catheterization lab. I'm staying because this is surreal. Because this is the most real. Because this is someone's heart.

BECAUSE GETTING AN air mattress for the person who has been hospitalized for three months matters more than any media placement, corporate grant, or distributor contract ever did.

I'M STAYING FOR the gift of purpose. Because every lab result I attempt to interpret, every illness I study, makes me wonder. And wondering, it seems to me, is the purpose.

BECAUSE SOMEONE HAS to hit *silence* on the IV pump alarm.

AT SUNSET, I glance at the building across the street and catch a reflection of the apartment beside mine. In looking out, I see within. They're seated around a table. A woman is laughing. The patient is laughing, just for a moment. I can't hear her. I'm looking out. I see events unfolding around me. I see that which encompasses me, but remains hidden. Just for a moment, I see how she might look at a dinner table. She's not wearing a gown. She's not bruised. I've never met my neighbors, but in looking out I see how close we are.

BECAUSE THERE ARE poles of fascination and repulsion, and between them is the point of maximal impulse. Because I fear apathy.

BECAUSE A PATIENT leaning against a wall in the hallway of 7W says she was told to stay away from her room but doesn't know for how long—the nurse spoke in English. The patient speaks Spanish. In English, the nurse explains to me that she simply told the patient to get a little exercise and gestured to the hallway. Of course the patient can return to her room now! Of course she need not stand alone in a gown with a fistful of paper towels to catch her vomit.

BECAUSE ONE SHIFT is a fast track through time zones. New vocabulary. New fear, new capability. Because it crosses every line, and the passage is enticing. Because it's a little dangerous, a little uncomfortable. Draining. Delicate. Excruciating. Lovely. Because it doesn't allow me to stop thinking.

BECAUSE I HAVE been in the bed, and beside the bed. Because I have waited. Because I believe any one of us could face the circumstances of those for whom we provide care, and we're much more similar than different. Because this is where the rhythm is loudest—*yes this yes this yes this yes this.*

BECAUSE IT RESIGNIFIES. *How are you?*

BECAUSE THERE'S NO map and no way to pack for certain journeys, so voyagers have nothing to do but worry. Because the bedside tray and call button become the whole world. Because wisdom, grace, and ferocity hibernate in each tired body. Because even when thumping, the heart is fragile.

BECAUSE WHEN I needed an ultrasound, the tech had to switch the attachment to see between my ribs, and the new attachment made small cuts across my back. Because when she couldn't get a good view of my spleen, she pushed the light closer to my skin and barked, *Are you sure the pain you feel isn't scabies? You have some little red marks here on your back!* Because when I explained to her that the red marks were from the plastic edges of the new attachment, she just said, *Oh.* Because when I asked if she'd looked at the CT scan and seen the abnormality on my spleen that sent me there in the first place, she said, *No, I guess I should do that.* Because patients are treated like this every day.

BECAUSE WHEN ILL and alone, we're all astray. Entwined, entangled. Because courage does migrate, and the people I work with, the people I've cared for, know how to pin it down. Because they inspire me.

BECAUSE THE SCIENCE is magical. A scan. A silvery snapshot, a house in motion, convergence of persistence and arrest. Because of the petals blowing in the breeze of an angiogram, the blush of contrast. The whisper of removal. Because the medicines know where to go and how to fortify that which has been depleted.

BECAUSE THIS MORNING was warm enough to leave home without a jacket. Seasons change. This is not a blessing, but being able to notice it is. Because boats have returned to their harbors, and there are people who can't see them.

Acknowledgment of Permissions

WE ARE GRATEFUL to the authors who have given us permission to include previously unpublished work in this anthology. We also thank the authors, editors, and publishers who have given us permission to reprint the following selections.

HOLLY ANDERSON. "My Nontraditional Choice." Reprinted from *Case in Point Magazine,* 2007.

ANNE CASTON. "The Good We Do," copyright 2007. Reprinted from *Judah's Lion,* Cider Press, with permission of the author.

MARK CLARKE. "Night Shift" is reprinted with permission of the author from *Night Shift,* Myrmex Press, 1999.

THEODORE DEPPE. "One on One with Dylan Thomas" is reprinted with permission of the author from *Cape Clear: New and Selected Poems,* Salmon Books, 2002.

PATTY SMITH HALL. "How I Found My Way Back" appears by permission of the author.

ANN NEUSER LEDERER. "Notes on a Nursing Home" was previously published in *Geriatric Nursing*, Jul/Aug 1983, Volume 4, Number 4, pages 224–227, and is reprinted here with permission of the author.

VENETA MASSON. "Winter Count" first appeared in *Clinician's Guide to the Soul—Poems on Nursing, Medicine, Illness and Life* by Veneta Masson (Sage Femme Press, 2008).

PAULA SERGI. "Home Visits" is reprinted here with permission of the author. The poem also appeared in *Intensive Care*, University of Iowa Press, and in *The Poetry of Nursing*, Kent State University Press, 2006.

ELIZABETH TIBBETTS. "A Nurse Reads *A Book of Luminous Things*" first appeared in *The Beloit Poetry Journal*, "Home Visit" in *The Spoon River Poetry Review*. Both are included in the author's book *In the Well* (2003), Bluestem Press, 2002 Bluestem Poetry Award.

SALLIE TISDALE. "Why I Like Dead People" was first published in "The Sun," and appears here with permission of the author.

Reader's Guide

1. "Once a nurse, always a nurse," says Teresa Kenas. Do you agree? What is it about nursing that makes it a special calling, even among helping professions?

2. After reading Veneta Masson's essay, reflect on what your own "Winter Count" might look like. What memorable events stand out for you in your own nursing history? How have those events shaped the course of your career?

3. Multiple writers who decided to leave their nursing jobs, including Holly Anderson and Jenna Rindo, describe stomach pains before work as an important sign that they needed to change professions. What others signs might suggest a nurse is in the wrong job or needs more support? Is it possible for someone to regain his or her ability to be a nurse once they've burned out, or can they never return?

4. Nancy Seale Osborne wonders if she could have walked the tightrope of marriage and career. What have you had to sacrifice for your career or for your family? Think about how working in the field of nursing made this more

or less difficult for you. How did it affect your decisions about your work, or about marriage or children?

5. The images of mother and nurse have both changed significantly since the 1950s, when some of these authors began their training. How have changing ideas about mothers paralleled some of the changes in nursing? Think about how the changing status of women has contributed to new roles for mothers and nurses. How might things continue to change over the next 50 years?

6. Several authors touch on the subject of empathy. Sallie Tisdale describes the feat that comes with "unbordered empathy," while Judy Schaefer says she became an empath on the day she became a nurse. Is empathy an integral part of nursing, or is it a dangerous trap nurses can fall into? How do you know when you're identifying too closely with a patient? How do you know when you're distancing yourself too much?

7. These authors came of age at varied times. How did Elizabeth Simpson's description of nursing in the 1950s contrast with today's experiences? What changes have made the job easier, or harder? If you could choose something to bring back from the days of 1950s nursing, what would it be?

8. Theodore Deppe writes about being forced to make a decision, and draws a connection to a patient who

hasn't been able to stop using drugs. What painful experiences have forced you to make a difficult decision? Some people need a painful experience in order to make a change. What if that painful experience could be life-threatening to a patient? Would you ever wish for this moment of reckoning, if you believed it might lead to a better life for your patient?

9. Sallie Tisdale writes that dead people make her aware of her own vitality. The close proximity to death is an inevitable part of working in medical care. Do you remember the first time you saw the body of a person who had died? How does that compare with how you feel now? What coping mechanisms do nurses develop to deal with death?

10. In his poem, Jim Cardwell sighs that "being 99.9 percent" right can cost him his career. And yet nurses are required to be sure about things that no one can be sure about. How do you cope with the uncertainty inherent in your profession?

11. Jenna Rindo eventually traded in her nursing cap for a teaching position. She writes that she could never adjust to the "uncertainties involved in critical hospital nursing." In what ways is nursing more inherently uncertain than teaching? Why do so many nurses become interested in teaching when they decide to make a career change?

12. Some authors describe seemingly unimportant encounters that end up being significant in their career paths. Andrea Vlahakis describes a young girl who one day hopes to be a nurse, while Jeanne Bryner describes a chance conversation on a bus. What small encounters moved you along your path? Were you aware of their importance at the time?

13. Sometimes nurses need a new dose of inspiration. Colleen O'Brien describes just such an experience on a trip to Alaska with her husband and young son. What experiences have helped inspire you during difficult times at work? To whom do you turn when your reserves are low?

14. Not all nurses become priests like Father Robert Kus, but many of the authors make reference to God when they talk about their work, or seem to see nursing as an inherently spiritual endeavor, like Anita Chupp. Do you feel there is a spiritual element in nursing? In what ways are nursing and ministering similar?

15. Colleen O'Brien depends on music as her "life source," and describes how she had to leave nursing and travel all the way to Alaska to find it. Other writers discovered their artistic calling as part of their nursing work. What is the connection between healing and art? What does it mean to find art as a nurse, or to leave nursing in order to purse the creation of artwork?

About the Editors

PAULA M. SERGI, BSN, MFA is the author of *Family Business*, a poetry chapbook from Finishing Line Press; co-editor of *Boomer Girls: Poems by Women from the Baby Boom Generation*, University of Iowa Press, and co-editor of *Meditations on Hope* and *A Call to Nursing*, both from Kaplan Publishing. The Wisconsin Academy of Sciences, Arts and Letters, along with the Hessen Literary Society selected her as the 2005 cultural ambassador to Germany for a three-month residency. A Wisconsin Arts Board Artist Fellowship recipient, her poetry appears in such journals as *The Bellevue Literary Review, Primavera, Crab Orchard Review, AJN,* and *Spoon River Poetry Review.* She has taught composition, fiction writing, and poetry at Ripon College, the University of Wisconsin, Oshkosh, and Marian University, and currently works as a school health nurse.

GERALDINE GORMAN, RN, PhD, is an Assistant Professor in the College of Nursing at the University of Illinois at Chicago. She holds an MA in English literature and a PhD in nursing, both from Loyola University, Chicago. Before coming to UIC in 2002, she taught at Western Michigan University. Prior to entering the nursing

256 *A Call to Nursing*

profession in 1991, she taught writing as a teaching assistant at Loyola University. She also worked in direct social services, living in community at the Little Brothers of the Poor and participating in all aspects of their service to low-income elderly, including meal delivery, relocation services, and holiday and vacation celebrations. In this capacity, she also facilitated poetry workshops in nursing homes, resulting in two small anthologies of collected work. She was a founding member of a small grass roots organization in Tempe, AZ, which served the needs of the many relocated elderly and she organized the local university community to provide, among other services, respite care for the spouses of Alzheimer victims. Before beginning nursing school, Gerry served as the volunteer coordinator and editorial assistant to H.O.M.E, a nonprofit housing organization for Chicago's low-income elderly.

About the Contributors

HOLLY ANDERSON completed her RN degree in Ft. Collins, Colorado. Her nursing experience includes working in the clinical setting as well as case management. Her background also includes working as an occupational health nurse for Universal and Warner Brothers Studios. She obtained certification in Case Management in 2006. She continues to work as an ambulatory case manager. She and her husband make their home in California.

MICHELLE ASHLEY received her BA in urban public policy and worked as a union organizer for nurses in California. She moved back to Chicago to study nursing and became an oncology nurse working at the University of Chicago. She currently works as a nurse case manager for uninsured women helping them gain access to free breast and cervical cancer screenings. She is also currently going to school for her Master's in Advanced Community Health Nursing at UIC.

LAURIE BARKIN, a psychiatric clinical nurse specialist, received her undergraduate and graduate degrees in nursing from Boston University. Recently, she completed a memoir about her work with surgical trauma patients at San Francisco

General Hospital during the 1990s. The major theme of the book is vicarious traumatization, focusing on the PTSD-like symptoms that caregivers may experience as a result of their exposure to others' pain and suffering.

SALLY BELLEROSE is a retired RN who was privileged to spend 20 years working with the amazing staff and individuals living with intellectual and physical challenges at Monson Developmental Center in Western Massachusetts. She is also a writer who has many awards including an NEA, The Barbara Deming Prize, and the Rick DeMartinis Award. Her recently published work appears in *Rock and Sling, The Journal of Humanistic Anthropology, Passager, Cutthroat, Crab Orchard Review, Cup of Comfort for Writers, Per Contra,* and *Saint Ann's Review.*

JEANNE BRYNER was born in Appalachia. Her books in print are *Breathless, Blind Horse,* and *Tenderly Lift Me: Nurses Honored.* She has received writing fellowships from Bucknell University, the Ohio Arts Council, and Vermont Studio Center. Her poetry has been adapted for the stage and performed in Ohio, West Virginia, Kentucky, New York, California, and Edinburgh, Scotland. Her book *No Matter How Many Windows* is forthcoming from Wind Publications in Kentucky.

JIM CARDWELL has been an RN for 30 years (24 in emergency medicine) and served as a Vietnam Corpsman. He is also a poet, folk musician, cowboy, and organic salsa grower/maker. His poetry and songs have been published by *The Acorn, Struggle, Poetalk, Cover, The Pegasus Review, The Journal of Nursing Jocularity, Cowboypoetry.com,* and more. He tours widely in the western states as a cowboy poet. His CDs of poetry/music include *A Son of California,* and *Five Silver Dollars.* A CD of nursing poetry/songs is being recorded now.

MARYLOU CARRERA is a nursing student at the University of Illinois at Chicago.

ANNE CASTON is a former nurse, now a writer and an educator whose work has been published in literary and medical journals here and abroad, and whose first collection of poems, *Flying Out with the Wounded,* was awarded the 1996 New York University Press Prize for Poetry. She has been a featured writer twice on WPFW's "The Poet and the Poem" and was interviewed by Michael Collier for *The Writer's Life* video series, broadcast over a tri-state television area (D.C., Maryland, and Virginia). Her work has recently been anthologized in collections such as *The New American Poets: A Bread Loaf Anthology, Where Books Fall Open, Sustenance & Desire,* and *Long Journey: Contemporary Northwest Poets.* A selection from Anne's poems was awarded Prairie Schooner's 2002 Readers' Choice Award and her poem "Purgatory" received an International Merit Award in Poetry from *Atlanta Review.*

ANITA CHUPP is a nursing student at the University of Illinois at Chicago.

MARK H. CLARKE lives and works in Chico, California. He entered the nursing profession as a second career in 1992. While earning his Bachelor of Science degree, he developed a passion for writing. His poems have appeared in the journals *Watershed* and *California Quarterly;* others have been anthologized in *This Little Bit of Earth,* and *The HeArt of Nursing.* He currently works as Administrative House Supervisor and Clinical Educator at Enloe Medical Center in Chico.

THEODORE DEPPE has 20 years of experience in intensive care and psychiatric nursing. His books include *Children of the Air* and *The Wanderer King* (Alice James), *Cape Clear: New and Selected Poems* (Salmon), and *Orpheus on the Red Line* (Tupelo, 2009). He teaches in the Stonecoast MFA program and directs Stonecoast in Ireland. He has been a writer in residence of the James Merrill House (Stonington, CT), the Poets House (Donegal), and Phillips Academy (Andover, MA). His awards include two NEA grants and a Pushcart Prize. A dual citizen of the U.S. and Ireland, he presently lives in Galway.

WILLIAM DINEEN is a nursing student at the University of Illinois at Chicago.

JULIETTE AST DOLS is currently completing a Master's degree in nursing at the University of Illinois at Chicago to become a midwife and nurse practitioner. In addition to being a student, Dols also serves as an RN at University of Chicago's labor and delivery, and as a research assistant at UIC's College of Nursing. A native of Wichita, Kansas, Dols moved to Chicago after completing her bachelor's degree in English literature at the University of Kansas. She and her husband live in Chicago.

KELLY FITZGERALD is a nursing student at the University of Illinois at Chicago.

KATHRYN GAHL loves red lipstick, ballroom dancing, and vintage clothing. She has traveled widely, working as life model, waitress, tour guide, editorial assistant, staff nurse, camp nurse, columnist, teacher, and Director of Women's and Children's Services. Now, she writes. Her stories and poems appear in numerous journals, including the *American Journal of Nursing, Drumvoices Revue, Notre Dame Review, Permafrost, Pindeldyboz,* and *Porcupine Literary Arts Magazine.* Mother of five young adults, she lives in rural Wisconsin with her second and last husband.

KATHERINE SUZANNE HARRIS is a writer and registered nurse. Her essays about being a nurse have been published in a variety of nursing magazines including *Nursing Spectator* and *The American Journal of Nursing.* Her work was also featured in the anthology *21 Peaceful Nurses.* Katherine graduated for Smith College in 1994, where she studied women's studies and writing. She then got a nursing degree from the University of Massachusetts in 1998, and has been a maternity nurse ever since. Katherine lives in the pioneer valley of Massachusetts with her husband and two children.

CHERYL HERNDON is certified nurse midwife who exemplifies the definition of the word "midwife." Midwife means "with woman." Cheryl has made it her lifetime goal to be supportive of women. She is founder and president of Womankind Services, a resource organization committed to providing information to women in every area including physically, mentally, and emotionally. Cheryl has been in the medical community since 1986, working initially as a nurse and later as a nurse-midwife and a nurse-practitioner. She is also a gifted speaker and published author. She may be contacted at Cheryl@womankindservices.com.

ELIZABETH JANE HILL graduated in 1968 from Presbyterian University of Pennsylvania School of Nursing with an RN diploma, and later earned a BFA in Sculpture from the University of the Arts in Philadelphia in 1986. Exhibited nationally and internationally, her sculptures have received numerous reviews and awards. From 1996-2000 she lived in Scotland, making and facilitating giants puppets for community-based pageants. Community-based arts eventually led her back into nursing. She now lives in her childhood home in Collingswood, NJ, currently teaching at Pennsylvania Academy of The Fine Arts and working for Bayada Nurses in pediatric home care.

NINA HOWES is a nurse, a political activist, and a writer. Her stories have been published by University of Iowa Press; her plays have been presented off-off Broadway and at the NYC Public Libraries with Around the Block. She loves theatre and has performed and produced off-off Broadway.

TERESA KENAS is an internationally unkown essayist and fiction writer. In 1988, she left a career in nursing to explore other means of service, which have included flight desk operator, data entry clerk, market researcher, travel agent, game show production assistant, paste-up artist, executive assistant, retail clerk, entrepreneur, and published author. After making her home in seven different states and traveling extensively worldwide, she resides once again in her native New York, further refining her methods of service through caring for elderly family members. She is currently writing a book.

JOAN STACK KOVACH is currently the Nurse Director of McLean SouthEast, a 25-bed inpatient adult psychiatric unit. She has been a nurse for 34 years, working in the fields of pediatrics, psychiatric/mental health, and community health. For five years she wrote a regular column for the *BayState Nurse News* and has contributed articles to *Nursing Spectrum*. In addition, her writing appears in the books *Intensive Care: More Poetry and Prose by Nurses,* by Davis and Schafer (2003), *Peer Consultation in the Group Context,* by Shields et al. (1985), and *Keeping the Public Healthy,* by Jarvis (1985). She is currently at work on a book about the two years she lived with her family in Hungary, entitled *100 Mondays in Budapest.* She lives in coastal Massachusetts with her husband, the poet George Kovach.

LISE KUNKEL is currently a home care nurse in the Finger Lakes region of New York State, where she lives with her husband, Scott, and daughter, Zoe. With many remarkable people, she has worked as both a volunteer and as an RN in end-of-life palliation for 20 years. She has read and written poems for well over 40 years.

FR. ROBERT J. KUS, Pastor of St. Mary Catholic Parish in Wilmington, NC, was ordained for the Diocese of Raleigh in 1998. Fr. Bob received his doctorate from the University of Montana in sociology, his post-doctoral masters' degrees in psychiatric–mental health nursing from the University of Oklahoma, and his M.Div. from St. Meinrad School of Theology in Indiana. A former Associate Professor of Nursing at the University of Iowa, he is currently a writer for various Hispanic magazines and is a consulting faculty member at UNC-Wilmington and UNC-Pembroke.

PIAF LATHAM-WINTERGREEN is a nursing student at the University of Illinois at Chicago.

ANN NEUSER LEDERER was born in Ohio, and has also lived and worked in Pennsylvania, Michigan, and Kentucky. Her poems can be found in journals, anthologies, and her chapbooks *Approaching Freeze* (Foothills), *The Undifferentiated* (Pudding House), and *Weaning the Babies* (Pudding House). She has degrees in Anthropology and in Nursing, and is employed as an RN.

VENETA MASSON is a nurse and poet living in Washington, D.C. "Winter Count" was inspired by a short story of the same name by Barry Lopez and appears in *Clinician's Guide to the Soul* (Sage Femme Press, 2008), a collection of poems and art that illuminates nursing, medicine, illness, and life.

DIANA MOTT has been a nurse for 30 years. For almost half of them she has been caring for oncology patients, witnessing their joys and sorrows, often being humbled by their grace. In 2007 she earned a Masters in Fine Arts in Creative Non-Fiction and is working on a collection of essays. She lives in New York City with her husband and son.

COLLEEN O'BRIEN received a Bachelor of Science Degree in Nursing from the University of Portland in 1974. She has worked as a certified poison information specialist, a triage and advice nurse, a clinic nurse, a home health nurse, a school nurse, and a hospice nurse. Together with her husband, Chris Lee, she now performs in a contemporary chamber jazz duo called PrimalMates in which vibes, voice, cello, and percussion come together to form an inspired original repertoire. Their music features the attention to composition and form of chamber music with the freedom and improvisational interplay of jazz. In addition to voice, which she can use with words or as another instrument, she's known for her unusual approach in playing cello like a jazz bass and her spirited cello solos.

NANCY SEALE OSBORNE is a mother, grandmother, and great grandmother. Her intention upon her 1953 graduation from high school was to become a nurse, but she was requested to leave the Shannon School of Nursing program in San Angelo, Texas, because she got married in her first year of training. She thinks she would have been a good nurse and she values all of the nurses who completed their training and worked in the field. Nancy is Librarian Emerita, State University of New York College at Oswego. Her BS and MS are from that institution and her MLS is from the School of Information Studies, Syracuse University. Her motto is: "I'd rather be canoeing!"

JO ANN PAPICH is a graduate of Iowa State University with a BA in English. Later, she received an Associate degree in Nursing from San Juan College of Farmington, New Mexico, and worked as an RN for thirteen years. She was an oncology certified nurse and cared for cancer patients on a busy medical floor. Combining her degree in English with her career in Nursing, she now works as a medical transcriptionist from an office in her home of Farmington.

JENNA RINDO graduated with a BSN in 1987, and worked in pediatric special care for seven years at hospitals in Virginia, Florida, and Wisconsin. Currently she teaches English to Arabic, Hmong, and Spanish students, and has a Master's in Reading Education. Her poems and essays have appeared in *Frontiers: A Journal of Women Studies, Kalliope, Ars Medica: A Journal of Medicine, the Arts and Humanities, Mom Writers Literary Magazine,* and other publications. She lives in rural Wisconsin with her husband, blended family of five children, a small flock of Shetland sheep, Bantam chickens, and other less domesticated animals that howl at the moon.

BARBARA SAUVAGE has worked as an emergency room RN for the past 12 years; prior to that, she worked in hospice and med-surg nursing. She has read her pieces on the nursing experience at Hektoen Institute of Medicine Nurses and the Humanities programs, as well as the University of Illinois at Chicago's Humanities in Nursing Art Day performances under the direction of UIC's Dr. Geraldine Gorman. Previously published in UIC's *Penlights* anthology as well as the "Kaplan Voices: Nurses" anthology *Meditations on Hope*, she is married to Ken Sauvage; they have two wondrous daughters, Leah (married to the great Micah), and Genevieve.

JUDY SCHAEFER, edited the first biographical/autobiographical work of English-speaking nurse-poets, *The Poetry of Nursing: Poems and Commentaries of Leading Nurse-Poets* (The Kent State University Press, 2006), and co-edited the first international anthology of creative writing by nurses, *Between the Heartbeats* (University of Iowa Press, 1995), and more recently, *Intensive Care* (University of Iowa Press, 2003). She has published a collection of poems, *Harvesting the Dew,* (Vista, 1997), and has been published in journals such as *Academic Medicine, The American Journal of Nursing,* and *The Lancet.* Memberships include The Kienle Center, Penn State University, College of Medicine, and Sigma Theta Tau International Nursing Honor Society. She is the East Coast Editor for *Pulse: voices from the heart of medicine,* an e journal. Her website is judyschaefer.biz.

KELLY SIEVERS, a nurse anesthetist, lives in Portland, Oregon. In 1968 she graduated from St. Mary's School of Nursing in Rochester, Minnesota, a school of revered mentors. The sixties were a time of unrest and great changes in the United States. Our teachers persevered and entrusted to us the legacy of nursing: a reverence for the mystery of the body and a respect for it. Kelly's recent poetry is published in *Ratttle, Ekphrasis, Windfall, Prairie Schooner,* and two anthologies: *Vacations* (Outsider Press) and *The Poetry of Nursing, Poems and Commentaries of Leading Nurse Poets* (Kent State University Press).

ELIZABETH SIMPSON was born in Canada, and earned her Master's at the University of British Columbia. Her nonfiction work includes *The Perfection of Hope: Journey Back to Health* (M&S, 1997), Spanish translation, nominated for B.C. Book Prize and VanCity Book Prize, and *One Man at a Time: Confessions of a Serial Monogamist* (M&S, 2000), nominated for the VanCity Book Prize. Her short stories include "Dressed for Suicide" (CBC, 2002), "Puppy Love" (CBC, 2003), and "Slipping the Noose" (*Matter of Choice,* Seal Press, 2004). Her novel *Under the Marmalade Moon* is currently being considered for publication. Her biography *The Literary Atlas* was published by Greenwood Press. Elizabeth also serves as a reviewer for *The Globe and Mail* and *Monday Magazine.*

PATTY HALL SMITH, the research director for Neuropathy Solutions, writes devotionals and Christian fiction. With articles in *Guideposts, Journey,* and multiple newspapers across the country, she was recently awarded the Genesis Award by American Christian Fiction Writers for her historical romantic fiction. She lives in Caledonia, Michigan, with her husband, Dan, and their two daughters, Jennifer and Carly.

KATHLEEN WALSH SPENCER practices in post-anesthesia nursing. She is former editor-in-chief of *Plastic Surgical Nursing*, has written dozens of articles for the nursing literature, and works for the Center for Health Research at Wayne State University. Her poems have appeared in *Clackmas Literary Review, Rosebud, Red Rock Review*, and other journals, as well as in the collection *Intensive Care: More Poetry and Prose by Nurses*, and a chapter in *The Poetry of Nursing: Work and Commentary by Major Nurse Poets*.

SHIRLEY STEPHENSON is an ER nurse and writer. Prior to becoming a nurse she worked as a communications and development professional with an International healthcare organization and a Chicago-based arts organization that promoted creative literacy in public schools. She has received an Illinois Arts Council Artists Fellowship and her writing has appeared in various literary journals. She is currently studying to become a family nurse practitioner.

CARISSA SWIATEK graduated with a BA in English from Colgate University, and will receive her BSN from the University of Illinois at Chicago in 2009. She lives in Champaign, Illinois, with her husband and dog.

ELIZABETH TIBBETTS works on a medical-surgical unit, and has worked in a variety of settings during her nursing career. Her book of poems *In the Well* (2003) won the Bluestem Poetry Award. Her poems have appeared in journals such as *The American Scholar, Green Mountains Review,* and *Prairie Schooner,* and have been nominated for *Pushcart* and featured on *The Writer's Almanac.* She lives in Maine.

SALLIE TISDALE's most recent book is *Women of the Way: Discovering 2500 Years of Buddhist Wisdom* (Harper, 2006). Her essays and stories appear in *Harper's, Antioch Review, Tricycle,* and other magazines.

ROYCE JANE UYECHI graduated from Texas Women's University in 1965 with a BS in Nursing. She taught Med-Surg at Lillie Jolly School of Nursing in Houston, Texas. After working part-time in various Med-Surg settings, she returned to full-time work as a school nurse with the Northside ISD in San Antonio, Texas. She retired from school nursing and is now doing telephonic nursing as a Health Coach in Denver, Colorado.

ANDREA VLAHAKIS is an RN, writer, and teacher. Her poems have appeared in *American Journal of Nursing* and *Intensive Care: More Poetry and Prose by Nurses* (University of Iowa Press), among other publications. Her nursing experience includes oncology, acute care, and pediatrics. She is also a children's writer. Her picture book *Christmas Eve Blizzard* was the ASPCA Henry Bergh Children's Book

Award Finalist. She lives, writes, and teaches writing for children in Connecticut.

In 25 years of hospital nursing, **ANNE WEBSTER** held positions in Critical Care and Nursing Administration. Her work has recently appeared in *The Poetry of Nursing: Commentaries and Poems of Leading Nurse Poets* and *Rattle*. *A History of Nursing,* her poetry collection, is forthcoming from Kennesaw State University Press.